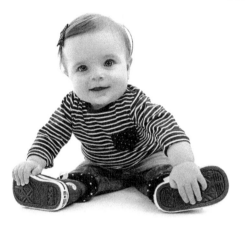

BURNS, FALLS AND EMERGENCY CALLS

The ultimate guide to the prevention and treatment of childhood accidents

"Arm yourself with Emma's great book, take sensible precautions and then let your children enjoy their childhood"

Dr Amanda Gummer
The Good Toy Guide

Helping you keep children safe, from birth to adulthood

Emma Hammett

Visit www.firstaidforlife.org.uk and www.onlinefirstaid.com
for updates and free resources

9030 00001 4448 7

Published by First Aid for Life

All rights reserved. No part of this publication may be reproduced, stored in a retrieval system or transmitted in any form or by any means electronic, mechanical, photocopying, recording or otherwise, without the prior permission of Emma Hammett or the publisher.

Burns, Falls and Emergency Calls has been written by Emma Hammett, qualified nurse, first aid trainer and founder of First Aid for Life and onlinefirstaid.com in conjunction with other medical, first aid, health and emergency services professionals.

The contents are based on the Resuscitation Council UK guidance, European Research Council guidance on First Aid (ERC) and ILCOR (International Liaison Committee on Resuscitation) recommendations. The information is current at the time of publication and will be reviewed and updated with new editions.

Disclaimer: the author has made every effort to ensure the accuracy of the information contained within this book and whilst the book offers guidance it does not replace medical help. The author does not accept any liability or responsibility for any inaccuracies or for any mistreatment or mis-diagnosis of any person or animal, however caused. If you suspect illness or injury, you should always seek immediate professional medical advice.

The photos on the covers are credited to Ben Barlow Venture Studio Milton Keynes. The picture is Florence (Emma Hammett's great niece).

Burns, Falls and Emergency Calls
The ultimate guide to the prevention and treatment of childhood accidents

Children don't come with manuals or on/off buttons. They will have minor accidents and that is normal and healthy. This book is designed to prevent the big, scary accidents, to help parents and child carers become more aware of potential risks, to teach the skills needed to help in an emergency, and ultimately to save lives.

As an experienced nurse and first aid trainer, I have seen time and again how important prompt and appropriate first aid is in those first few minutes following an accident. Yet so many people still lack the vital skills needed to make a difference when it matters most.

Not only does immediate first aid save lives, it can also reduce pain, suffering and make a dramatic difference to the speed and extent of a child's recovery. Understanding how to treat an injury or illness yourself and feeling confident identifying when something is serious can also save you many unnecessary hospital visits.

I established First Aid for Life in 2007 and it has grown steadily to become a multi award-winning practical and online first aid training business. Our training has equipped thousands of carers, parents, teenagers, sports/health professionals and caring members of the public with the skills and confidence to help in a medical emergency. My motivation for founding First Aid for Life came from treating a little boy in the burns unit who was so badly scalded he needed skin grafts. Had someone given him basic first aid, he probably wouldn't have needed to be admitted to hospital. First aid treatment is so simple, and knowing what to do could have saved that little boy so much pain and scarring.

As a mother and member of a huge, close family, I continually use my first aid knowledge and am forever grateful that I can quickly judge how seriously hurt or ill someone is and know the best way to help. This has enabled me to calmly administer first aid to my family at home and saved countless unnecessary trips to hospital.

Burns, Falls and Emergency Calls is a clear, accessible reference guide showing you how to help if your child, or a child you care for, is involved in a medical emergency. This book is designed for parents, teachers, childminders or anyone working with or caring for children.

The content of this book is supported by our practical first aid training (www. firstaidforlife.org.uk) and our online courses (www.onlinefirstaid.com), both of which help to make first aid skills more accessible to everyone. There are lots of helpful free resources and courses available on both these sites.

Acknowledgements

I would like to thank my family and friends for all the incredible support they have given me with First Aid for Life. Thank you for posing as injured casualties, humouring me in my never-ending search for perfection, and for always being there when I need you.

Thank you to my superb team of trainers and administrative support, who continually inspire me with their passion, expertise and loyalty. Special thanks to Adriana, my incredible graphic designer in Buenos Aires who created all the fabulous illustrations for me.

Thank you too to my amazing customers, who continue to give such wonderful feedback and prompt me to push boundaries to enable more people to benefit from these skills.

This book is dedicated to all of you.

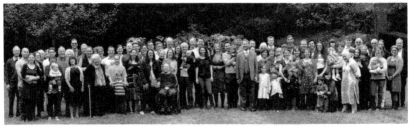

The ultimate guide to prevention and treatment of childhood accidents

Contents:

Foreword

Introduction

How to use this book

PART 4: Useful information

PART 5: Resources

Forewords

"Children have an unnerving knack of taking their parents and carers by surprise. Emma's book places safety in the context of child development, empowering parents to anticipate risk and avoid serious accidents in childhood. She shows how prompt first aid can help minimise the impact of an accident, sharing her practical knowledge and skills. And she explains how to assess a situation, so we have the confidence to apply first aid skills in an emergency."

- Katrina Phillips

Chief Executive, Child Accident Prevention Trust

"Being a parent is scary and we have a natural tendency to over-protect our children. Rather than wrapping the children in cotton wool, arm yourself with Emma's great book, take sensible precautions and then let your children enjoy their childhood. Being armed with the knowledge and skills to deal with accidents is much more practical than trying to foresee and prevent every mishap."

- Dr Amanda Gummer

MD & Founder

The Good Toy Guide, Good App Guide and Fundamentally Children

"'Burns, Falls and Emergency Calls' is a pleasure to read and written using Emma's decades of experience in nursing and first aid. Parents, carers and anyone working with children and young people will appreciate the way that Emma has focused on child development accidents and injuries, as well as outlining the norms of developmental expectations for different age groups. This unique and informative book is a must."

- Laura Henry

Award-winning international Early Years specialist.

"Children are curious and it's only natural that they will have minor accidents as they explore. 'Burns, Falls and Emergency Calls' is a super informative, but easy to read book, for families, parents, grandparents, childminders and carers, to help everyone become aware of potential risks. It teaches the skills needed to help in an emergency without overwhelming the reader, and of course, that could ultimately save lives. This great book empowers and gives confidence to everyone who reads it and I highly recommend that you go out and grab yourself a copy and keep it handy."

Sue Atkins

ITV 'This Morning' Parenting Expert & Author of 'Parenting Made Easy'

– How To Raise Happy Children

www.TheSueAtkins.com

Introduction

The health and happiness of children in our care is of vital importance to us and we always do our best to keep them safe. However, every year around 2 million children attend A&E due to an accident. Over 100,000 of these require admission to hospital – that is nearly 2,000 children a week.

150,000 people die every year in situations where first aid could have saved them. Accidents are second only to cancer as the leading cause of death for children and young people in the UK. You never know when something might happen. Prompt and appropriate first aid saves lives, and can reduce the severity of injuries and speed recovery.

Children need to take measured risks, from which bumps and bruises will inevitably result. This is normal and healthy. However, it is important to prevent serious childhood injuries that can cause long-term damage and have life-changing consequences. The part of the brain that evaluates risk and consequence is not fully developed until the early 20s. Therefore, it is vital for parents and those working with children to be aware of potential dangers and to equip themselves and the children with the knowledge and skills to keep themselves and others safe.

This book is designed to help you anticipate the next developmental milestones for your child (from birth right through to adulthood), and take the necessary measures to prevent life-threatening injuries and mishap.

How to use this book

Burns, Falls and Emergency Calls is packed full of practical hints and tips relevant to different age groups. I have drawn upon my personal and professional experience and examples from friends and colleagues to introduce real-life tips and anecdotes.

The information contained within this book should help give you the confidence to:

- Anticipate developmental milestones and take precautions to prevent possible injuries
- Calmly approach any injury or medical emergency
- Assess the severity of the situation
- Quickly prioritise if there are any life-threatening injuries
- Reassure the sick or injured hild and treat the most urgent issues
- Seek medical advice or call an ambulance if necessary

The most important advice of all is to stay calm. If you are panicking, the casualty will pick up on this it will make things worse. Stress and panic will exacerbate any symptoms of shock, make breathing problems worse and mean it's much harder to help.

- The underlying principles of first aid are to:
- Preserve life
- Prevent further injury
- Promote recovery

Basic first aid is about using what you have around you, employing simple skills and improvisation, to do the best you can for the casualty.

This book is written to the latest guidance from Resuscitation Council UK and the European Resuscitation Council. However, first aid techniques and advice are continually under review. Please refer to our website which is packed full of free resources which are continually updated and will include the most up-to-date first aid information. We would also recommend you consolidate your learning by joining us for a practical or online first aid course.

Keep this book easily accessible and revisit sections at regular intervals to ensure your knowledge stays fresh.

PART 1

PRIORITISING INJURIES AND CHILD SAFETY

Recognising when something is seriously wrong and when to call an ambulance

When someone has an accident or is ill, it can be difficult to assess how serious it is and whether it's necessary to call an ambulance.

The following information aims to help you with this extremely important decision; the answer will vary from case to case, but I would strongly advise you to administer first aid and call an ambulance if the casualty:

- Doesn't appear to be breathing, is having chest pain, is struggling for breath or is breathing in a strange way, for example, appearing to 'suck in' below their rib cage and using other muscles to help them breathe.

- Has a severe injury that is bleeding profusely and won't stop, even when direct pressure is applied to the wound

- Is unconscious or unaware of what is going on, experiencing weakness, numbness or having difficulty speaking.

- Has a fit for the first time, even if they seem to recover from it later. It is important to phone an ambulance if someone has a seizure which lasts more than three minutes.

- Has a severe allergic reaction. It is important to administer their adrenaline auto-injector (if they have one) and then phone an ambulance immediately.

- Is seriously burnt. For a child or an elderly person with a burn severe enough to need dressing, put the burn under cool running water and call an ambulance. Keep cooling the burn until the paramedics arrive and look out for signs of shock. For a fit adult with a burn, cool it under water for at least 10 minutes – longer if it is still hurting badly – then apply a burns dressing or loosely cover with cling film and transfer them for immediate medical attention.

- Has fallen from a height, been hit by something travelling at speed (like a car) or been hit with force whilst doing combat or contact sport and there is a possibility of a spinal injury. If they are conscious, keep them completely still and get an ambulance on the way. If they are on their back, unconscious and breathing and you are concerned about their airway, very carefully roll them into the recovery position and phone an ambulance. If they are unconscious and not breathing, start CPR. If you are on your own and treating a child, do CPR for one minute before phoning for an ambulance.

Take someone to A&E if they have:

- A fever and are floppy and lethargic
- Severe abdominal pain
- A cut that is gaping or losing a lot of blood, an amputated finger or if they have something embedded in a wound
- A leg or arm injury and can't use the limb
- Swallowed poison or tablets and are not showing any adverse effects (111 can give you advice from the poisons database). If someone has swallowed something poisonous and is behaving strangely/experiencing other symptoms, call an ambulance immediately.

Go to your family doctor for other less serious and non-life-threatening medical concerns. Contact your GP or phone 111 for medical advice.

How to phone an ambulance

Phoning an ambulance is something people assume is second nature. However, in a highly stressful situation, it is easy to find your mind has gone blank. Emergency telephone numbers are different worldwide; you'll get through to the emergency services operator in the UK with 999 and with 112 throughout Europe. The number is 911 in the USA and 000 in Australia. They will ask you which service you require – police, fire or ambulance.

The operator will need to know exactly where you are, so use reference points, landmarks, ask locals or use google maps and give as much information as you can to help them to establish your exact location.

Use speaker phone so you can continue to provide first aid treatment whilst talking to the emergency services. Do what they advise.

They will need to know:

- Your name

- The telephone number you are calling from

- Your location (including postcode if possible)

- The type of accident

- The number of casualties

- The approximate ages of casualties

- Whether the casualties are conscious, unconscious and breathing, or not breathing

- Any other relevant information (such as whether they are taking medication)

If it is a life-threatening emergency, tell the emergency services immediately.

The emergency services will want to work through their algorithm of questions in order to classify your call. If your call is serious, they will already have despatched the ambulance, but still need to collate all the information to feed through to the medical responders.

Child developmental stages and recognising risk

Children develop at different rates: they reach milestones at totally different times and some miss out stages altogether. You will know your child well, but may not anticipate at what point they will suddenly roll, become mobile or be able to reach new heights.

The Child Accident Prevention Trust conducted a survey in 2012 with 2,700 parents and found that:

• Almost one in four were regularly taken by surprise at their child's ability to do something they thought they couldn't.

• More than half said they had been taken by surprise in the past.

It is exciting to see how quickly children grow and develop, and to revel in new developments such as them grabbing things, rolling over, crawling, standing, climbing, opening bottles and turning handles. However, it's when these new abilities take us by surprise that they can lead to serious childhood accidents.

The purpose of this book is to reduce the element of surprise and enable you to enjoy new achievements, having planned ahead and prepared for any threats to a child's safety.

When my children were younger, we had regular visits from older cousins and friends' children. This gave us some insight into the next stages for our little ones. Things of no interest to our children, or things way out of their reach, became a source of fascination for our visitors. Anticipating possible risks was incredibly useful as it meant we were always one step ahead in the battle to stay safe!

The following information outlines patterns of child development and will give you an overview of the next stages for your child, or children you are looking after.

Babies: from birth to crawling

Babies do not come with instructions. They are all different and bring unique challenges. Hormones and sleep deprivation combined with parental exhaustion and the responsibility of a tiny new baby can be totally overwhelming, particularly for first-time parents.

With a new baby comes an irrepressible need to protect them and make them happy. You'll be overwhelmed by scare stories, conflicting information, advice and an endless list of do's and don'ts!

Fortunately, young babies are fairly well-designed and don't get up to too many dangerous exploits, so the risk of accident is relatively low. Most young babies admitted to hospital have either respiratory infections or have had an accidental fall, usually whilst being carried to or from bed.

New born baby characteristics:

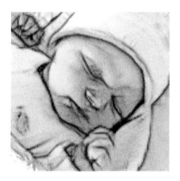

•   A large head in relation to body size, which makes them head-heavy.

•   A soft-spot or fontanel on top of their head – this will fuse together in the first 10–18 months

•   Very thin, sensitive skin – 15 times thinner than an adult's

•   Bendy bones and a flexible rib cage

•   Very little control over their own movement

•   A strong grasp reflex

•   Can kick, wriggle and wave their arms

3 months

•   Babies may be able to roll over independently from front to back, or back to front

•   Grabbing things

•   Put things in their mouths

6 months

- Many babies can sit up unsupported

- Push and pull things and roll to get to things

- Many babies begin to crawl or move in some other way independently

One of the major parental fears is Sudden Infant Death Syndrome (SIDS). This is now included within the umbrella term SUDI – Sudden Unexpected Death in Infancy.

SIDS

Sudden Infant Death Syndrome (SIDS) is the sudden and unexplained death of a baby where no cause is found after a detailed post mortem.

Every year in the UK, 300 babies die suddenly and unexpectedly in their sleep due to Sudden Infant Death Syndrome (SIDS). This statistic sounds alarming, but SIDS is rare and the risk of your baby dying is low.

While there is no advice which can guarantee the prevention of SIDS, there are recommendations for parents and carers to reduce the risk to their baby:

- The safest place for a baby to sleep for the first six months is in a cot, Moses basket or crib in their parents' room.

- Avoid your baby spending too long in a car seat, or sleeping in a semi-upright position. Transfer them to their cot or Moses basket as soon as possible.

  Current advice is not to leave your child in a car seat for more than 30 minutes.

- Place your baby to sleep on their back on a firm mattress that is in good condition, with their feet at the foot of the cot, to avoid them wriggling under the covers.

- Do not cover your baby's head.

- Don't let your baby get too hot, ideally the temperature in the room should be between 16°C and 20°C.

- Falling asleep with a baby significantly increases the risk of SIDS if the parent is a smoker, under the influence of drugs or alcohol, or just extremely tired.

- Parents can reduce the risk of SIDS by not smoking while pregnant or after the baby is born.

- Breastfeed your baby if possible.

Most deaths happen during the first six months of a baby's life, but these recommendations are relevant for the first 12 months. Infants born prematurely or with a low birthweight are at greater risk. Babies with a parent or parents who smoke are in a far higher risk category.

Weaning

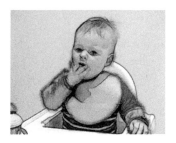

Many parents are apprehensive about starting their baby on solids and rightly worried about choking. Babies do have a very sensitive gag reflex. Often, they have alarming facial expressions and can make frightening noises when they are just experimenting with new food textures. Gagging is a normal reflex, choking is not.

The choking section of this book will explain how to recognise the signs and help if your baby is choking.

Most common accidents

- Falls from raised surfaces, baby bouncers, high chairs and down stairs.

- Suffocation from bed covers, in baby slings, from nappy sacks.

- Choking on food or small objects.

- Strangulation from ribbons, blind cords, drawstring bags hung over the cot.

- Poisoning from carbon monoxide.

- Burns and scalds from hot drinks, bath water, sunburn.

- Drowning - babies can drown in a couple of centimetres of water.

Safety advice for babies

Never leave babies unattended on a raised surface or in the bath, not even for a second.

> *I have seen many cases in hospital when a baby left on the table in their bouncy chair has managed to bounce themselves onto the floor. Tables are a long way up and floors are usually a hard landing.*

Nappies are best changed on the floor as there are so many cases of babies who have rolled off the changing table in the split second their parent has reached for something.

- Never place bouncy chairs or car seats on a raised surface.

- Always strap your babies into highchairs and buggies.

- Ensure you hold onto the banister when carrying your baby downstairs.

- Fit safety gates to your stairs before your baby starts crawling.

- Do not use duvets and pillows with babies under 12 months.

- Babies should sleep on their back in the feet to foot position.

- Keep nappy sacks and small objects well away from babies - if they grab them they can easily suffocate as they don't have the dexterity to remove them from their faces.

- Keep pets away from small babies.

- Don't leave toddlers and other young children alone with your baby.

- Never hang drawstring bags on cots, avoid cot bumpers which tie around the cot and use blind cord clips or alternatively choose a cordless blind.

- Fit a carbon monoxide alarm and have appliances regularly serviced.

- Don't drink hot drinks whilst holding a baby, and never pass hot drinks over a baby's head.

- Be careful of microwave hot spots when heating bottles and food - always shake or stir thoroughly and test the temperature before feeding the baby.

- Fill a bath with cold water first and use a bath thermometer as well as checking the temperature yourself before bathing the baby.

- Never place a cot by a radiator.

- Use strong factor baby sun cream in the summer.

- Keep babies in the shade, wear UV protective clothing and hats, and avoid midday sun.

Babies - crawling to walking

At this age, babies are mobile, inquisitive and keen to explore. This is when you need eyes in the back of your head, as they always seem to navigate towards inappropriate and potentially dangerous things. This is where you find them eating cat litter, or poking things in their ears or up their nose.

> *It is not usually a medical emergency if someone has something in their nose or ear, but you do need a health professional to remove it safely. Numerous times in hospital we have needed to extricate bits of eraser, toys or food from various orifices. Once we even found a sprouting pea!*

Many babies don't actually crawl, but find an alternative way of shuffling on their bottoms to get from A to B. Some walk or climb without ever bothering to crawl.

Characteristics of babies from 6 months to toddling

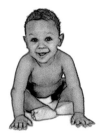

- Large heads in proportion to their bodies - still head heavy
- A propensity to put everything in their mouths
- Unsteady, whether sitting or mobilising

- Eating solid food, chewing and biting with new teeth
- Pulling themselves up on things
- Opening and shutting things, trying to fill empty objects and posting things through gaps
- They don't learn from experience

From around 12 months, babies learn that objects out of sight still exist and they may try and climb for things put out of their reach.

Some of the most common accidents for this age group are:

- Falls from stairs, windows, chairs, cots and highchairs.

- Suffocation from bedding, plastic bags and nappy sacks, packaging.

- Choking on food and other objects.

- Internal injuries from button batteries, cleaning products and dishwasher tablets being swallowed.

- Strangulation from clothing, ribbons and necklaces, blind cords, or something hung over their cot.

- Poisoning from tablets, cleaning products, plants and anything else they can get their hands on and put in their mouths.

- Burns and scalds from kettles, hot drinks, hair-styling equipment, radiators, bath water and the sun.

- Drowning in baths, paddling pools, swimming pools.

    Babies can drown in as little as 2cm or so of water.

- Amputated fingers from hinges and slamming doors.

- Bumped heads as they stand up under things, walk into things and bump heads with other children.

- General bumps and bruises, cuts and grazes as they fall over whilst exploring.

Safety tips for this age group

- Fit stair gates and keep stairs clear from clutter.

- Teach your baby to come down the stairs backwards.

- Always hold the stair rail when going up or downstairs

- Never leave chairs next to a window, work surface or somewhere dangerous that your baby can climb to.

- Strap them into the buggy and highchair.

- Nappy changing is always safest on the floor.

- Keep plastic bags and packaging out of reach and dispose of them carefully.

- Always stay with your child when they are eating or drinking.

- Discourage older children from sharing their food with the baby.

- Keep small items and all batteries well out of children's sight and reach.

- Never put necklaces or dummies round a baby's neck.

- Do not hang drawstring bags over the cot, tie blind cords out of reach.

   Strangulation from children climbing and slipping with their head through a string or cord is not uncommon in this age group.

- Medicines should be locked away; a childproof container may only delay them getting at them!

- Be careful with bags or handbags left on the floor, they may have numerous potentially lethal hazards inside.

- Lock away household detergents, buy dishwasher capsules or tablets rather than granules as they are marginally less damaging if swallowed and choose cleaning products containing Bitrex which is bitter to discourage children from swallowing it.

- Keep hot drinks out of reach, use a kettle with a short flex and keep it at the back of the work surface.

- Use the back rings of the cooker, turn pan handles away from the edge.

- Always stir food and drink to avoid microwave hot spots.

- Fit a thermostatic valve to the bath to avoid temperature surges, run the cold tap first and use a bath thermometer.

- Fit fireguards and radiator guards, turn off heated towel rails.

- Be particularly careful of irons, hair straighteners and other hot implements and keep them and their flexes well out of reach when cooling.

- Never leave a baby or child alone in the bath, even for a second.

- Supervise water play at all times and always empty paddling pools and bowls of water immediately after use.

- Be very careful with ponds and swimming pools.

- Use soft corner covers for hard and sharp corners.

- Use door stops to prevent doors slamming.

- Secure furniture to the wall with furniture straps to prevent it toppling if a child tries to climb on it.

- Baby walkers have been the cause of numerous accidents and are not recommended.

- Always adhere to the recommended age ranges on children's toys.

It is of the utmost importance that children are put in the appropriate car seat and buggy for their height and weight. Contact a reputable dealer for the latest advice and take advantage of their fitting service to ensure your child is protected while travelling.

A cup of tea is still hot enough to scald a baby 15 minutes after it has been made.

> *It was a little boy, scalded by a cup of coffee that inspired me to start first aid for Life. His mum panicked when she spilt hot black coffee over his arm and the side of his head and rushed outside screaming for someone to help. Had she calmly run the affected area under cool running water, his burns would undoubtedly have been less severe and he may not have needed skin grafts.*

> *Always check everywhere else that a hot liquid could have splashed. We looked after a baby who had hot tea spilt over him. The main injury on his arm was treated under cool running water, but the tea had soaked into the baby's Ugg boot; no one had realised and his foot was very badly burnt.*

Toddlers: one to three year-olds

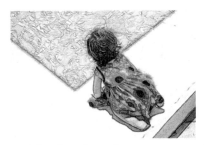

This is the age you really do need eyes everywhere! These guys are fast, strong-willed, stubborn, headstrong and completely devoid of any form of risk awareness; a totally lethal and truly exhausting combination.

They have boundless energy, a total lack of awareness of the consequences of their actions and little fingers they can poke into just about anything.

Characteristics of one to three year-olds

- They are still head heavy, with large heads compared to the rest of their body

- Thin, delicate skin

- Flexible bones that are still developing and growing

- Pretty good dexterity to remove screw tops, open door handles and climb up to get to things that are out of reach

- A short attention span

- An inability to gauge exactly where sound is coming from and therefore identify possible danger from oncoming traffic etc.

By fourteen months

- They may be able to walk without help and possibly run.

- They may be able to crawl upstairs.

- They can cause havoc with your cooker, TV or anything else that is appealing. They often become obsessed with knobs, dials and switches and are very good at posting things through gaps or poking things in spaces.

When my son was little, we searched high and low for the knobs from our cooker, only to find them posted down the back of the sofa! He could so easily have choked on them, so be vigilant.

By two years

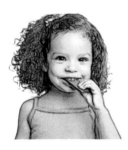

- Still put everything in their mouth

- Explore the taste, smell and texture of objects and may put objects in any orifice!

- Will begin to copy adult behaviour

- Can open taps and screw tops

Some of the most common accidents for this age group are:

- Falls from windows, down stairs, from balconies, highchairs, buggies and off furniture.

- Injuries from falling furniture or bookshelves as they reach or climb to get something attractive.

- Suffocation from plastic bags and packaging.Choking, particularly on food, but also small toys, coins and sweets.

- Choking, particularly on food, but also small toys, coins and sweets.

- Strangulation. Be particularly careful with blind cords, clothing, necklaces and drawstring bags on doors, hooks, handles or over cots.

- Poisoning from dishwasher tablets, cleaning products or tablets.

- Burns and scalds from hot drinks, bath water, sunburn, radiators, hair straighteners, irons, oven doors and fireplaces.

- Drowning in the bath, swimming pools, ponds, buckets and the sea.

- Cuts, bruises, crushed and amputated fingers and bumped heads.

The paramedics in my team have told me about an alarming rise in the number of injuries resulting from overloaded buggies. The issue arises when there's a child in the buggy and a child on a buggy board at the back, as well as shopping hanging on the handles. If the child in the buggy suddenly gets up, the buggy is catapulted backwards and the child on the back will whack their head hard on the floor behind. Don't hang shopping off the handles as it is unsafe and will cause the buggy to tip.

Safety tips for this age group

Toddlers fall over repeatedly, run into things and stand up underneath things. They seem to be obsessed with everything inappropriate and potentially dangerous.

Stair gates can be helpful, but be careful as your little one gets older; they may start to see them as a challenge that encourages them to try and climb them or play with the catches, and this can be dangerous. Safety gates are not recommended for children over 24 months, but judge the situation based on your own child - remove the gate or change its position as soon as your child can climb or open it. Fitting the gate on the landing or bedroom door can be a safer option than at the top of the stairs. Parents should be careful with safety gates too as we frequently see accidents due to parents trying to climb the gates.

Children this age are naturally inquisitive and will climb on anything, so be careful of pot plants and chairs by windows and on balconies. Every year we hear of miracle escapes when a child has fallen from a block of flats or out of a top floor window - sadly not every child is so lucky.

The CAPT has recommendations on safe gap widths for open windows and the spacing for balcony railings and stair banisters. 6.5cm (2.5") is recommended until 18 months. A larger gap of 10cm (4") has been introduced for 18 months and older as most children's chest widths exceeds 10cm so they're unlikely to be able to squeeze through anything this size.

Advice for this age group

- Secure furniture - particularly bookcases, chest of drawers and TVs - to the wall. They can easily topple and crush a child if they're climbing up them.

- Always supervise children when eating. Chop fruit and vegetables, particularly grapes and avoid chopping into neat circles which can fully obstruct the airway if they get stuck.

- Keep small objects out of reach of children and ensure you adhere to the recommended ages for toys.

Button batteries are a particular risk for children this age as they tend to put everything in their mouths.

Button batteries and lithium coin batteries are small, round, batteries you find in toys, cards, watches, key fobs and numerous other everyday objects.

Lithium coin batteries are particularly concerning as they can burn through tissue and blood vessels within hours. Often parents are oblivious to the fact that their child has swallowed the battery and the first symptom they are aware of is their child vomiting blood. Sadly, this is often too late to save the child as irreparable damage has already occurred.

Sometimes, button batteries do pass through the body without a problem. However, if a battery gets stuck, energy from the battery creates corrosive caustic soda and it is this that burns through tissues.

If children pop a battery up their nose or in their ear, this can also result in lasting damage.

Prevention and vigilance is key

- Always check battery compartments are securely fastened.

- If a battery is missing and you think your child may have swallowed it, take them to A&E for an x-ray.

- Store and dispose of batteries carefully, out of children's reach and sight.

If you think your child may have swallowed a button battery - act fast!

Take them to your nearest Accident and Emergency department immediately.

- Do not wait for signs or symptoms

- Do not try to make them sick

- Do not give them anything to eat or drink

Your child will be x-rayed and, if necessary, be taken for an operation as soon as possible to remove the battery.

- Try and prevent your toddler accessing the bathroom or loo alone as this is often where tablets and loo cleaner are found. Children often like playing and flushing things down the loo.

- Be careful to keep things both out of sight and out of reach. Poisoning is a particular problem at this age. Children are incredibly inquisitive and will eat or drink anything they fancy. Child-resistant packaging is not childproof and only slows them down a bit. Be careful around the house and garden too; particularly as seasons change, the garden becomes a new area to explore and a place to find unexpected hazards!

- Discourage children from eating any plants in the garden or countryside.

- Also be extremely careful when visiting other people, particularly grandparents, who may put their medication in obvious places so that they remember to take it. The contents of Granny's handbag, or that of any visitor, could prove lethal too!

- Make sure you fit, and regularly test, carbon monoxide alarms.

- Keep hot drinks out of reach and remember that a drink made 15 minutes previously can still burn a child even if it's at drinking temperature for an adult.

- Use a kettle with a short flex, and put pans at the back of the cooker. Be careful not to inadvertently encourage children into dangerous behaviour by drawing up a chair for them to stand on and reach the cooker. Consider putting a safety gate to restrict access to the kitchen when cooking.

- Fit a thermostatic mixing valve to bathroom taps to prevent heat surges if another tap is used. Put cold water into the bath first.

- Always apply appropriate sun cream (re-apply after swimming), cover up and keep children out of midday sun.

- Use fireguards and radiator covers. Switch off heated towel rails as they become incredibly hot and are usually at child height. Children don't necessarily know to let go if they are burning. Keep irons, hair straighteners and any other hot appliances and their cords well out of reach.

- Never leave children unattended in the bath or near water even for a second. Children can drown in a couple of centimetres of water. Always empty water play immediately after use. Cover water butts and garden bins. Be extremely vigilant at swimming pools, around ponds and at the beach.

- Children this age are prone to poking their little fingers into hinges and around doors and often crushed fingers and even amputations result. Door stops and hinge strips are helpful in avoiding these injuries.

- Keep children clear of the buggy when it is being folded and don't let them play with bike chains.

> *One of my friends was in hospital having her second baby. Her husband was at home with their toddler and they were just preparing to go out. He went to open out the buggy; put his foot on the bottom to push down and did not realise that his toddler's finger was in the mechanism. The little boy's finger came off! Little fingers and toes can be amputated in anything with a hinge. Keep clear of bicycle chains too.*

- Keep scissors, knives and razors well out of reach.

Children should not be left alone in cars, even when strapped in. When travelling in cars, they should be in a car seat appropriate to their weight. It may be prudent to fit a play tray to their car seat and have toys available to distract them from trying to fiddle with the clip and attempting to release themselves from their car seat. Ensure child locks are activated on the cars to prevent them accidentally opening the door.

> *My brother fell out of the car in a car park when he was little and had a very narrow escape!*

Three to five year olds

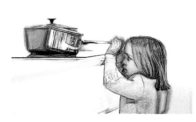

At this age, children are keen to copy adult behaviour. They have very short attention spans and can become frustrated very quickly. They are headstrong, stubborn and generally unaware of risk and danger unless it is spelt out to them.

They will begin to learn that their behaviour can affect others and that leaving toys on the stairs for example could lead to someone else having an accident. However, they may not remember this fact when they're in the middle of a game or adventure.

Characteristics of this age group

- Children are beginning to understand cause and effect and that there can be consequences to their actions. They have improving co-ordination and dexterity and can open and reach more things.

- They still have short attention spans and are not interested in simple safety instructions.

- They are easily distracted and led and are implicitly trusting.

- Role play is important to them and they are often totally absorbed in their imaginative games. They may take on a totally new persona as an animal or made-up character.

- They are likely to use toys and play equipment in kinds of ways never intended by the manufacturer.

- They are becoming increasingly sociable.

Most common accidents for this age group include:

- Falls down stairs, from windows, balconies, playground equipment, bunk beds and other furniture.

- Choking.

- Strangulation, particularly from blind cords.

- Poisoning.

- Burns and scalds from hot liquids, candles, radiators, hot water, sunburn.

- Drowning - be particularly vigilant near swimming pools and by the sea.

- Cuts, bruises and bumps to the head.

- Falling off bikes and scooters.

Safety tips for this age group

- Remove safety gates at this age as children are likely to see them as a climbing opportunity, which causes accidents.

- Teach children to hold banisters and go steadily up and down stairs.

- Fit safety locks to windows and do not place furniture or plant pots near windows or on balconies where they can provide something for the child to climb onto.

- Bunk beds are not recommended for children under 6.

- UK Electrical sockets have additional safety mechanisms and it isn't easy for children to force things into them and electrocute themselves. Socket covers can damage UK sockets and are no longer recommended.

- Always supervise children when eating. Discourage them from running around or talking whilst eating.

- If they are eating a lolly, they should be sitting down and not running around with a lolly stick sticking out of their mouth.

I have seen many horrible accidents resulting from children falling over or off bikes or trikes with a lolly in their mouth - it can go right through their soft palate!

- Poisoning is a big risk for children of this age. They will be able to swiftly break through childproof containers and cupboard catches. If you are staying with relatives, they may quickly find tablets and contraceptive pills.

One of my friends found both children with an empty bottle of paediatric paracetamol. Both were taken to hospital for urgent treatment. A paracetamol overdose can cause permanent damage to the liver. It is vital to keep all medication well out of sight and reach.

- Berries are also tempting for this age group, so be particularly vigilant, particularly at Christmas time as many ornamental winter plants are extremely poisonous.

- Always clear up on the evening of a party. Otherwise your children may be the first downstairs in the morning and ready to consume any dregs and leftovers.

The Christmas rose causes such bad diarrhoea that it was used as a chemical weapon by the ancient Greeks.

- Children this age like to copy adults. They will want to help cook, light can-dles and can turn on taps, heaters and electrical appliances such as irons and hair straighteners. They will be aware that these things get hot, but will not realise how hot until they have burnt themselves.

- Remember that fancy dress costumes are not usually flame proof. Be particularly careful near any naked flames.

Claudia Winkleman's daughter was out trick or treating and brushed against a candle on the doorstep. She caught alight and her fancy dress costume and tights melted onto her, causing appalling injuries.

- Fit a thermostatic bath tap to prevent temperature surges and ensure children never climb into the bath until you have checked the temperature. Always run cold water first.

- Apply appropriate sunscreen, and re-apply after swimming. Avoid the midday sun.

Keep hot drinks out of reach and never pass a hot drink over someone's head.

- Children do not have the skills to safely cope with traffic until they are much older. At this age, they should not be allowed to cross the road on their own.

- Children should start being taught basic safety. Explain why things are poisonous or dangerous rather than telling them not to touch etc.

- When booking children into Children's Activities, ensure the Activity Provider has all the necessary safety elements in place. Ideally choose an Activity Provider regulated by the CAA (Children's Activity Providers' Association) or an equivalent awarding organisation.

Five to 11 year olds – primary school

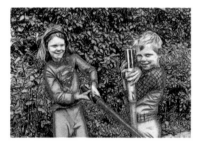

By the age of 5, most children are sociable and easily influenced. It's at school that they begin to realise not all adults parent in the same way. It is at this age that you may start to hear "it's not fair!" and "Joe's mum lets him do it!"

They may join clubs and outside activities and begin to be exposed to new safety challenges. Play is still of great importance and many will enjoy role play, making things and sports.

There is very little in terms of dexterity that a child of 7 upwards can't manage. Child resistant packaging presents minimal challenge. They are generally good at understanding danger, but remain impulsive and excitable and may well forget to be careful. They also frequently over-estimate their own abilities.

Adult supervision and guidance remains critical to prevent accidents, particularly if younger siblings are around. Boys are more disposed to injury than girls.

The sense of adventure may lead older children in this age group to want to play in unsuitable and unsafe places such as railway lines, building sites and in derelict buildings.

Nothing is totally inaccessible to older primary school children; they usually find a way of getting to things they want. Therefore, it is vital to equip children in Years 5 and 6 with the tools to evaluate risk and to explain that they are now role models for younger children at primary school. It is good for children at the top of the school to have mentoring roles supporting some of the younger children. It is great preparation for secondary school and helps them start to develop a sense of independence.

Characteristics of this age group

- Good dexterity and fine motor skills

- A tendency to over-estimate their abilities

- Increasing levels of independence

- Quick reactions, being fast, headstrong and impulsive

- Ability to use scissors, tools, kitchen implements and play with toys that contain small parts. These can present a potential danger for younger children.

Most common accidents for this age group include:

- Burns and scalds

- Choking - usually from food and sweets

- Falls - particularly from play equipment

- Drowning

- Cuts and bruises

- Road accidents

Safety tips for this age group

Children will want to copy adults and are likely to want to help in the kitchen. Supervise children closely if they are involved with anything to do with hot food and drink. Matches, candles and lighters can be fascinating for children but they also present major risks.

I looked after a little boy on the burns unit who had been playing with his brothers in the sitting room. They were playing with matches and set fire to the heavy curtains that landed ablaze on top of this little lad. He was in hospital for months and will bear the scars for life.

Children should always sit when eating. Deter them from chatting and running around whilst eating to avoid choking. Encourage them to sit down when eating lollies - I have seen many horrendous accidents from children falling whilst enjoying a lolly, forcing the sweet through their soft palate.

Children will explore and play games on equipment which pushes it beyond its original design. Most play equipment is well designed and serious injury is rare. However, it is important to point out if specific inappropriate use could prove dangerous. Children should keep clear of swings when they are in use and be encouraged to hold on when attempting challenging feats -injury often results from showing off!

Supervision is still necessary near swimming pools, lakes and in the sea. Currents in the sea can be extremely strong for a young swimmer. Teach them to recognise the flag system for safe swimming on supervised beaches.

Road safety is also incredibly important. Children should be taught the Green Cross Code - to stop, look and listen. Extra care should be taken with the increasing number of silent electric powered vehicles. They should be taught to look out for bicycles and motorcyclists travelling between lanes.

One of my son's friends was crossing the road sensibly looking left and right, but was hit by a bicycle going at speed up the middle of the road. He was temporarily knocked out and ended up needing an ambulance.

Children should always wear helmets when cycling. There are excellent cycle safety schemes to start teaching safer cycling. Younger children in this age group should not be cycling on roads in traffic. If children are going to be cycling to secondary school, then they need to learn safe cycling to be ready to do this.

Eleven to sixteen - secondary school

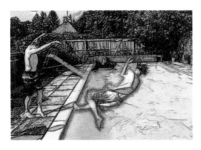

Peer pressure is incredibly important at this age and teenagers are classic risk takers. Dares can become increasingly inventive and dangerous and can involve persuading each other to do extraordinary things. Bullying can also be an issue, so look out for signs and try to keep open and non-judgemental communication with your teenagers.

Eating round a table is even more important at this age as it is a great time to catch up and ensure things are going okay at home and school.

Parents are no longer taking children to school and back and may feel distanced from the school life. You may not know your children's friends or their friends' parents. The first sleepovers can be daunting for a parent and, yes, it is perfectly acceptable to phone the friend's parents (despite the outcry from your child). Likewise, it is sensible to phone when they are going to parties to ensure that there will be adult supervision and understand the stance on sleeping arrangements, alcohol and under-age drinking. Ensure your child understands the effects of alcohol and how vulnerable it can render them. Ensure they know how to help someone who has drunk too much.

Children this age often look to push boundaries. The sense of danger can be perceived as a challenge and so think carefully how you raise the subject.

- More than 532,000 young teenagers have been left to cope with a drunken friend who was sick, injured or unconscious in the last year.

- A third of teenagers have had to cope with someone with a head injury.

- One in five teenagers has had to help someone who is choking.

- A quarter of young people have had to deal with asthma attacks.

Crucially: when faced with these emergency situations, 44% panicked and 46% simply didn't know what to do.

In the survey's most compelling statistic, 97% of young people believed first aid education would improve their confidence, skills and willingness to act in a crisis. *Source - British Red Cross*

> *When he was 14, my son and two friends were wine waiters for someone's 18th. Everything was going well, the parents were at home (although upstairs), but the teenagers were getting drunk at the party. Suddenly they discovered a lad unconscious outside (it was October) and the 18-year-olds were totally out of their depth. It was my son and his friends who helped to bring him back inside, checked he was breathing, covered him to keep him warm and rolled him into the recovery position. The older kids were desperate not to let the parents know, but it was the sober 14-year-olds who realised how serious this was -they were the ones who phoned an ambulance and got the parents from upstairs.*

Alcohol severely impairs someone's ability to regulate their body temperature and they can quickly develop hypothermia.

> *On her Duke of Edinburgh expeditions, my daughter had to help both a friend experiencing an acute asthma attack and another suffering from heat exhaustion.*

> *One of the teenagers who attended our courses went home and saved his dog's life with the first aid skills he learnt. It was this that led to the birth of our sister company, First Aid for Pets.*

Characteristics of this age group

- Increasing independence, increasing exposure to alcohol and drugs which makes them more vulnerable.

- Their friends are of vital importance to them and parents are not cool! Peer pressure and fitting in is critical and they may consequently do daft things.

- They are impulsive, sociable and not risk aware. They feel they are totally invincible and have everything ahead of them. If something does go wrong and they are out of their depth, they unravel quickly and need parents or a responsible adult to help quickly.

Most common accidents for this age group include:

- Sporting injuries - breaks and sprains

- Falls, head injuries, cuts and bruises - assaults (boys more than girls)

- Drowning - sea, open water swimming, swimming pools

- Burns and scalds - sunburn, hot drinks and beauty appliances

- Road and transport accidents (more boys than girls)

- Poisoning - alcohol and drugs

- Self-harm (more girls than boys)

Teenage boys are three times more likely to be hospitalised for transport related accidents and assault than girls. Girls are three times more likely to be hospitalised for self-harm.

Experimenting with drugs and alcohol makes teenagers far more vulnerable and unable to fully assess, comprehend or react appropriately to risk or danger.

Safety tips for this age group

- Teenagers should be encouraged to undertake an online or practical first aid course. This will encourage them to be more risk aware as well as equipping them with the skills and confidence to help themselves and others in an emergency. My children have both had to use their first aid skills on numerous occasions both on themselves and their friends.

- Sport should be in a supervised environment. When playing contact sports, you should never continue playing following a concussion and should follow all the latest recommendations and guidance concerning sport and head injuries. There is a section on concussion and sport later in this book. Always use protective equipment. Mouth-guards, helmets and shin pads should be compulsory if relevant to the sport.

- Talk to your teenager about safe drinking. Explain what alcohol does to your body and brain. Advise them not to drink on an empty stomach and to pace themselves - shots are not sensible. Help them understand the warning signs if they have drunk too much and to ensure they are in a safe environment with friends and don't end up in a compromising situation.

- Testosterone and alcohol combined can often lead to fights. Anyone who has been drinking and has a head injury should be checked by a medical professional.

- Help your teenager understand the consequences of diving into shallow water. They should always enter water feet first if they are unsure of the depth. They should never swim alone and always be supervised if swimming in the sea or open water. It is dangerous to swim after drinking alcohol. Diving into extremely cold water can cause a cardiac arrest.

- Look out for any indication of self-harm, bullying or depression in both boys and girls. Keep open lines of communication and encourage them to tell you how they feel.

- Always ensure you know how your teenager is getting back from a party. Be prepared to collect them and ensure they know they can call you whenever and wherever and you will help them in a non-judgemental way. Any questions can be answered in the morning when everyone is safe and sober. Always ensure they have the means to get home by taxi should you be unable to get them.

In our house, the rule is if your phone battery is down to 3% you need to come home. Since we instigated that condition, our children have become far better at taking a back-up charger and being more responsible about keeping in touch. If plans change, I expect a text. I need to know where they are going, what time to expect them back or where they're staying. Providing I have that information, there is mutual respect and trust.

Try not to nag! I am the worst culprit for it as it can be extremely difficult and frustrating to parent teenagers. However, just let them know you love them and will be there for them whatever.

Seventeen and up - college, sixth form, driving and independence

Characteristics of this age group

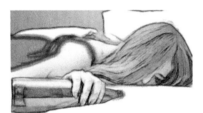

- Independent
- Private
- Sociable
- Strongly influenced by their peer group

Many of this age group are driving and are new drivers with very little experience of different road conditions. They may be driving friends and could easily be distracted. Their mobile phone is vitally important to them and they must understand how dangerous it is to make phone calls when driving.

The first time living away from home is a major learning curve.

Most common accidents for this age group include:

- Overdoing the alcohol, plus repercussions from this such as accidents, head injuries, grazes, trips, falls and brawls.

41

- Burns and scalds in the kitchen and from hot drinks.

- Cuts from learning to cook and fend for yourself.

- Transport accidents from driving, cycling and as a pedestrian.

Safety tips for this age group

- If they are learning to drive, go to a reputable driving school and encourage them to learn over a long period of time, rather than try and pass as quickly as possible. Arrange a motorway driving test once they have passed their test and supervised driving in different driving conditions, such as night driving, pouring rain, snow and ice to ensure they are confident in a range of different driving experiences.

- Speak with them about evaluating risk when accepting a lift from a friend who has only just passed their test. What is the driver like?How long has it been since they passed? How long did they learn for? Weather conditions? Is it a night or daytime journey? Are they using country roads or motorways? Who else will be in the car?Where are they going or coming back from?

- If they are going to festivals, ensure they are aware of potential risks and are with sensible friends who will look out for them. Encourage them to pre-book a locker so they will be able to charge their phones and deposit valuables (and back-up money) in there safely. Make sure they are pitching their tents somewhere sensible, no one is smoking anywhere near their tents and ensure they have appropriate footwear and clothing.

- Prepare your child with the skills to cook and fend for themselves; teach them both cooking and safety in the kitchen. Ensure they have good safe knife skills and are aware of the importance of food hygiene, sell by and use by dates.

- Encourage them to wear helmets and high visibility jackets or bands when cycling.

When is it safe to leave them home alone?

The law doesn't state an age when you can leave a child on their own, but it is an offence to leave a child alone if it places them at risk. Use your judgement on how mature your child is before you decide to leave them alone, whether this is at home or in a car.

The National Society for the Prevention of Cruelty to Children (NSPCC) states:

- children under 12 are rarely mature enough to be left alone for a long period of time

- children under 16 shouldn't be left alone overnight

- babies, toddlers and very young children should never be left alone

Parents can be prosecuted if they leave a child unsupervised 'in a manner likely to cause unnecessary suffering or injury to health'.

How old should a child be before they can babysit?

People can be prosecuted for neglect if they leave children on their own and something goes wrong. This is a highly contentious issue and one that becomes even more complicated when looking to establish when a child is old enough to be left in charge of other children.

When asking an older sibling or friendly teenager to babysit, it is vitally important to consider how competent they would be in an emergency. Ask yourself:

- How mature and responsible are they?

- Are they familiar with your home and any risks within it?

- How well do they know your children and do your children know and feel safe with them??

Remind your babysitter to be particularly careful of hazards including hot drinks, pets, tiredness and anything else that could cause a danger. You should explicitly point out these things as potential dangers so they understand that it's a responsible job.

Would an older sibling be a better option?

Research published in 2010 in Injury Prevention, a BMA journal, revealed that when older siblings supervise younger children, there is an increased risk of injury. Mothers tend to spot and remove dangers, whereas older siblings often interact with hazards, for example, making a hot drink and leaving it accessible.

Older children may resent being asked to look after siblings and so everything should be handled sensitively. Children also took more risks when being supervised by sibling, copying what they were doing and failing to listen when being told off. This led to an increase in accidents and injuries.

A babysitter is entrusted with another child's life and that is a tremendous responsibility.

The following preparation when you are using babysitters will lead to a safer arrangement:

- Ensure your babysitter is first aid trained.

- Fully brief them, introduce them to your children and familiarise them with your home.

- Remind them they are there to supervise your children safely and adhere to your rules.

- Have a local back-up adult available.

- Make arrangements in advance for the sitter's safe return home.

- Complete an emergency check list, available from our website.

- The babysitter needs to know:

    - Your children's names

    - Dates of birth

    - Allergies or medication

    - Your mobiles and work telephone numbers

- GP contact details

- Emergency telephone numbers (999/112)

- Reliable neighbours' numbers and addresses

- Location of electricity and water mains

Parents need time away. Most babysitters are good, and the children stay safe and happy. However, it does no harm to think carefully and plan before leaving them; everyone will be that much safer as a result.

PART 2:

LIFE-THREATENING EMERGENCIES

The second section of this book is about how to help if something does happen. It takes you through step by step, explaining how you should approach someone following an accident. It then guides you through recognising if someone has a life-threatening emergency.

How to help in an emergency

The first few minutes following an accident are often the most important, but also the most frightening for the first person on the scene.

It is important not to rush in. Take a deep breath, ensure the situation is safe for you and then calmly approach the casualty, speaking to them as you go. If there is more than one casualty, assess the quiet ones first as anyone making a noise is likely to be breathing.

Managing an incident

- **Assess the situation and make safe.**
- **Give emergency aid.**
- **Get help.**
- **Deal with the aftermath.**

You should always start by checking for danger - especially if you don't know what has caused the injury. If you're injured too, you won't be able to help them.

You need to keep yourself safe the whole time. Keep doing a dynamic risk assessment to ensure you don't put yourself in danger at any point.

KEEP AS CALM AS POSSIBLE

ALWAYS KEEP THINGS AS SIMPLE AS YOU CAN. TREAT WHAT YOU SEE!

Consent

A first aider should ask for consent, prior to giving treatment to a casualty.

If someone is unconscious, then consent is presumed under common law and the first aider is at liberty to help them in order to save their life.

If the casualty is a child, consent should be sought from their legal guardian prior to treatment being given. If the parent/legal guardian is not present, you should consider what is in the best interest of the child and act accordingly.

However, keep in mind that it is not for you as a first aider to impose your will on anyone else. If the casualty doesn't wish to be treated, keep yourself safe, step back and contact the emergency services from a distance. Explain the situation and pass the responsibility on to the ambulance crew who can arrange to have the patient sectioned under the Mental Health Act if they believe their refusal to accept treatment might cause death or serious injury.

Priorities of treatment

The key objectives of first aid are to:

- Preserve life
- Prevent the condition worsening
- Promote recovery

When you are dealing with a serious incident, it is crucially important that you prioritise any life-threatening conditions and treat those first.

Breathing is your number one priority. If they are not breathing and you don't do anything about it, they will die!

Bleeding and **burns** are both potentially life-threatening conditions.

Provided that the casualty is breathing, your next priority is to stop bleeding and treat burns before being distracted by anything else.

If the amount of blood being lost is extremely serious, known as a catastrophic bleed, this will take priority over breathing and it should be a priority to control the blood loss as quickly as possible in order to save the casualty's life.

Broken bones are rarely life-threatening and can prove a distraction from more serious priorities.

Preparing for an emergency

Things to think about before something happens

It is very helpful to think in advance about how you would manage a medical emergency.

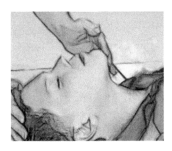

Make sure you have a fully-charged mobile phone with you and have close neighbours' numbers pre-programmed as well as those your next of kin. The ICE (In Case of Emergency) function on phones is extremely helpful and should be initiated on everyone's phones. Swap keys with neighbours and have their details in case you have an accident at home and need their help.

- Have a child's medical records easily available and take them with you in a medical emergency. **Do not delay going to hospital if these are not to hand.**

- Know where the electricity and water mains are located and how to switch them off. Ensure there are sufficient fire alarms, carbon monoxide sensors and a fire blanket.

- Know where the first aid kit is located - there should be a family one in the house, something smaller when you are out and about, and another kept in your car.

Find out where the nearest hospital is and what specialties they have. Learn where the out-of-hours chemist is situated and have their telephone number and opening hours to hand.

A few minutes on Google can readily supply you with these numbers and they should then be written up and placed prominently by the phone, so that if anyone else is looking after your children, they will have that information to hand. It is useful to have this laminated as a credit card sized document and keep it with you, should something happen when you're out.

In schools, nurseries and other workplaces

The Health and Safety (First-Aid) Regulations 1981 require employers to provide adequate and appropriate equipment, facilities and personnel to ensure their employees receive immediate attention if they are injured or taken ill at work. These regulations apply to all workplaces including those with less than five employees and to the self-employed.

What is 'adequate and appropriate' will depend on the circumstances in the workplace. This includes whether trained first aiders are needed, what should be included in a first-aid box and if a first-aid room is required. Employers should carry out an assessment of first aid needs to determine what to provide.

The regulations do not place a legal duty on employers to make first-aid provision for non-employees such as the public or children in schools. However, the Health and Safety Executive strongly recommends that non-employees are included in an assessment of first aid needs and that provision is made for them.

Further guidance can be found about making adequate provision for first aid in first aid at Work: The Health and Safety (First-Aid) Regulations 1981 - Guidance on Regulation.

- Ensure everyone knows the number to dial for the emergency services.
- First aiders and location of first aid kits should be communicated to staff and signs put up to remind people.
- An appointed person will need to be assigned to maintain first aid kits.

- Appropriate training needs to be co-ordinated and refreshed to ensure everyone is adequately trained for their responsibilities.

It is important that you keep as calm as possible. Keeping calm and avoiding panic has been shown to make a huge difference to the recovery of children, particularly if they are showing signs of shock, choking or are having an asthma attack.

- Assess the situation quickly and call for help swiftly if necessary.

- Keep yourself and others safe, remove any dangers, protect yourself and others and minimise the risk of infection.

- Prioritise casualties and injuries - treat the most serious first.

- Children should be transported to hospital with an adult they know and trust, and accompanied by a favourite toy or comforter if possible. This person should remain with them until their parents arrive. It is particularly important that children are helped to keep calm and reassured, as stress can make many illnesses much worse.

- If the accident is in a remote area, someone should be despatched to meet the emergency services and guide them to the casualty.

After the emergency:

- Clear up. Ensure you safely clean up and remove any body fluids that could be a hazard. You should hygienically dispose of contaminated items in a yellow incinerator bag or sanitary bin.

- Remove faulty equipment or anything else that could pose a danger to others.

- Ensure that appropriate paperwork and accident forms are completed.

- Restock anything that has been used from the first aid kit.

- Ensure that everyone is okay afterwards - dealing with a medical emergency can be extremely stressful and some people need professional help and counselling following such an episode. This is particularly important if children have been present and have witnessed the incident.

It is perfectly normal to feel any of the following after the event:

- A feeling of elation and an adrenaline buzz

- Anger

- Confusion

- Flashbacks and bad dreams

- Depression

If you're concerned, seek support.

The primary survey - how to help in an emergency

The primary survey is a fast and systematic way to find and treat any life-threatening conditions in order of priority.

Danger

Response

Airway

Breathing

Circulation/CPR

Danger

Check for electrical cables, broken glass, chemicals and make sure you do not put yourself at risk.

If the casualty is a stranger, approach with caution.

If there is any danger, remove it. If the casualty is being electrocuted, the electricity should be turned off at the mains before they are touched. Otherwise you could be electrocuted as well. If the danger cannot be removed (fire, flood, danger of explosion, chemical spills etc.) remove the casualty. Otherwise keep them where they are to avoid additional injury.

Make sure that everyone is safe. You are of no help to anyone if you become an additional casualty. Ensure any other children in your care are safe and if they are not casualties, delegate their care to another responsible adult so you can concentrate on the first aid.

Response

Once you're sure that the area is safe, you need to establish whether the casualty is conscious or not:

1. Shout assertively and ask them to open their eyes – see if they react in any way.

2. If there is no response, gently but firmly shake their shoulders or pinch the nailbed on their fingers or their ear lobes.

3. For a baby you can gently scrape the bottom of their foot with your fingernail.

4. If you get any response at all, you know they are breathing and their heart is beating.

5. If there is hardly any response and they are drifting in and out of consciousness but you have to leave them, put them into the recovery position first.

6. If there are multiple casualties, the quiet ones take priority as they may be unconscious and need urgent treatment.

Assessing levels of response

Alert – Fully responsive and conscious

Voice – Responds to you when you speak or shout to them

Pain – Groans or responds in some way when you pinch them

Unresponsive –Not conscious enough to keep their own airway clear

Someone is classed as unresponsive if they do not react at all when you speak to them or give them a painful stimulus.

Most common causes of unconsciousness (unresponsiveness)

FISH SHAPED

Fainting

Inability to maintain body temperature/imbalance of heat (e.g. heat stroke, hypothermia)

Shock

Head injury

Stroke

Heart attack

Asphyxia – lack of oxygen caused by an airway blockage (e.g. suffocation, drowning, asthma, choking, strangulation, gas poisoning)

Poisoning

Epilepsy/fitting

Diabetes

If you are treating someone who is unresponsive, other than ensuring your own safety (for example, in the case of carbon monoxide poisoning), do not waste time trying to find out the reason they're unconscious. It is vitally important that you swiftly establish whether they are breathing or not and take the measures necessary to save their life.

Airway

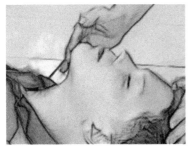

Tilt a child's head to a 'sniffing position'

When you are unconscious or unresponsive, most of your muscles relax and go floppy. Your tongue is a huge muscle attached to your bottom jaw. **If you are unconscious and lying on your back, your tongue will flop back and block your airway and you won't be able to breathe.**

In addition, your oesophagus (the tube from your throat to your stomach) and the sphincter (the valve) at the top of your stomach relax and remain open, so the contents of your stomach may trickle up and drip into your lungs. This is known as passive vomiting and is extremely dangerous to the casualty.

Note:

If someone is unconscious and you are aware of the presence of vomit because you can see it, smell it or they are gurgling, immediately roll them onto their side to empty them. If there is vomit at the back of their throat, they are unable to take a breath.

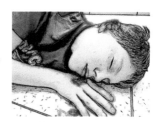

Passive vomiting

How to open someone's airway

Tilt the head and lift the chin. Try this yourself and you will find if your head is all the way back and you push your chin forward, you are unable to swallow.

By tilting their head and lifting their chin you are lifting their tongue from the back of their throat.

Never try and pull someone's tongue or put your fingers down to clear their airway. This is dangerous and could cause serious harm.

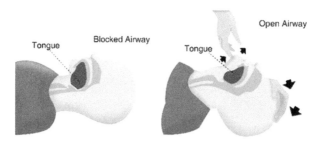

Put one hand on their head and the other under their chin and tilt their head back, lifting their chin upwards. This will lift their tongue away from the back of their throat so that their airway clears.

54

Note: ***For a baby, tilt their head and lift the chin to just horizontal. Do not over-extend a tiny baby's neck as you can bend their trachea, causing the airway to shut again.)***

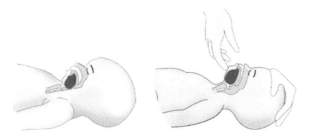

If the person is unresponsive and breathing, the only way to keep their airway open and clear is to put them on their side in the recovery position so their tongue will flop forward and any vomit drains from their mouth. (This is covered later in the book.)

Breathing

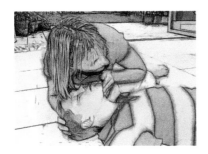

Just after their heart 'stops', a casualty may appear to be breathing when they are not. These breaths are called "agonal gasps" and are a reflex action from the lungs. Agonal gasps are not effective breathing. If there are fewer than 2 breaths in a 10 second period, the person is not breathing sufficiently and you will need to start CPR.

Hold the airway open and look. Listen and feel to check they are breathing. You need at least 2 breaths in a 10 second period to be sure that they are breathing normally.

- Tilt their head and lift their chin to open the airway and then place the side of your face above their mouth and nose and look down the body to check for breathing.

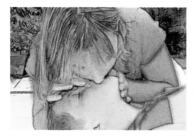 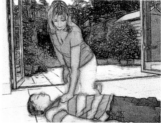

- Look for chest movements and listen for the sound of breathing.

- Feel their breath on your cheek.

If someone is unresponsive and not breathing normally, start **CPR.**

If in doubt, always start CPR - it is better to try and resuscitate someone unnecessarily than not to resuscitate someone who needs it.

For a child or baby start with 5 rescue breaths and then do 30 chest compressions – this will be covered in more detail later.

Unresponsive and Breathing

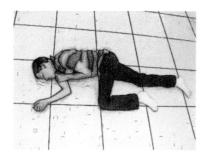

If the casualty is unresponsive and breathing normally, put them in the recovery position. The recovery position is putting someone on their side to allow gravity to help the tongue to flop forward and the contents of the stomach to drain out, to keep the airway clear and allow the casualty to keep breathing.

The casualty shouldn't be on their front as this would put the weight of their body on their lungs and it's not as easy to breathe. Therefore, with an adult or child, the knee is bent up at 90°, in a running position, to support them on their side. If the person has collapsed on their front and you are worried about a spinal injury, if you are sure they are breathing and their airway is not compromised, leave them as they are.

It is important that their head is turned sufficiently to allow saliva and vomit to drain forward. Providing you are not worried about a spinal injury, once on their side, tilt the head back slightly to further open the airway.

Once in the recovery position, keep checking that they're breathing; feel their breath using the back of your hand in front of their mouth.

How to put someone into the recovery position

The following method shows you how to put someone into the recovery position if you are on your own - even if you think they could have a spinal injury.

If you are not worried about a spinal injury, or if they are very heavy, you can just use their knee as a lever to propel them over into a draining position. If you are worried about the possibility of a spinal injury and you have other people to help, it is best to log roll them to keep the spine in line.

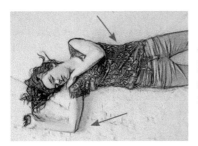

Move the arm closest to you out of the way. Use the hand closest to their head to hold their other hand and put this onto the side of their cheek to support the head and neck as you turn them.

Use your other hand to lift up the outside of their knee and use this as a lever to pull them over. Pull the knee to the floor, whilst supporting their head and neck with your other hand.

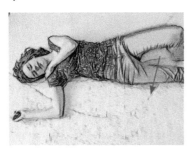 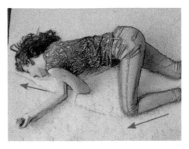

Pull their bent knee upwards into a running position to stabilise their body.

Ensure that they are over enough so that their tongue would be flopping forward and any contents of their stomach would drain out.

If you are not worried about a possible spinal injury, tilt their head back slightly to ensure the airway is properly open. If you are worried about a possible neck injury, just ensure they are rolled over enough to drain.

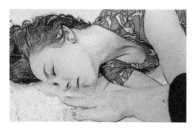

Keep checking that they are breathing by feeling their breath on the back of your hand. Get the emergency services on the way if they haven't already been called.

How to put a baby into the recovery position

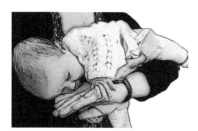

Option 1: Hold the baby in your arms, on their side, head lower than stomach. Use the back of your hand to feel their breath and keep checking that they are breathing. If you are unsure, wet the back of your hand as it makes it more sensitive. Call an ambulance.

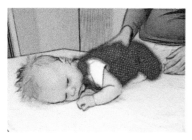

Option 2: Roll them into the recovery position on a blanket or coat to insulate them from the ground and use a rolled-up jumper or something to keep them on their side. Keep checking that they're breathing. Call an ambulance.

The secondary survey

Once the primary survey is complete and life-threatening conditions have been treated or are under control, it is now safe to conduct a secondary survey examination of the casualty, to establish if there are any other potentially life-threatening injuries you may have missed.

This is a detailed top-to-toe examination to discover what else is wrong and should only be undertaken if it is appropriate to do so. The casualty should be moved the absolute minimum necessary and if it causes them additional discomfort or stress, wait for the emergency services to arrive.

A secondary survey can be undertaken on a conscious or unconscious casualty. Either way, you should clearly explain the step-by-step process you are following and why you're doing it.

If someone is unconscious the secondary survey should be carried out with them in the recovery position and they should be moved as little as possible. You can conduct the secondary survey while waiting for the emergency services.
If there is any obvious core body or head injury, they should be placed onto the injured side.

Once they are in the recovery position and their airway is maintained, check for any other injuries, look for watery blood coming from either ear and feel their chest to see if both lungs are moving equally. Look for any other serious injuries such as bleeding or burns, or any other reason they may be unconscious.

Keep checking that they are breathing.

If the casualty is conscious:

Talk to them calmly and reassuringly and ask open questions to find out what is wrong.

Some useful questions:

History: ask what happened. This enables a proper assessment of the situation - to find out how the accident happened, whether they have hit their head or not and if there has been any short-term memory loss. It is also helpful to ascertain if there is any relevant medical history or medication that can be useful to tell the paramedics about.

Signs: What do they look like? Is there swelling, deformity of a limb; are they pale, cold, clammy, blue?

Symptoms: Where does it hurt most? This helps to work out exactly where they are injured. Can you take a deep breath? This helps to work out how seriously they are injured and whether their breathing is involved. It is particularly useful with children. When did the pain start? Does anything make it better or worse? How are they feeling? Useful answers could be along the lines of sick, dizzy, hot, cold, or thirsty but do not suggest any of these symptoms to a casualty; leave them to volunteer them.

Top-to-toe examination: Only do this if it doesn't cause any additional stress to the casualty. Most important information can be gleaned from looking and speaking with them, without needing to touch them at all. The paramedics will examine them properly as soon as they arrive.

If there might be a safeguarding issue or a crime has taken place, only examine them further in this way if you feel there may be a life-threatening injury you have missed.

If it is appropriate to examine them further, ask their permission to do so. Protect their dignity, keep them warm and explain what you are doing and why. Move them as little as possible. Wear disposable gloves to protect yourself from any blood or body fluids.

Protecting the airway is the priority. Do not do anything that could make things worse. If they are unconscious or losing consciousness and you are worried about their airway, they should be put into the recovery position straight away.

You are not a doctor! However, you are looking for any other potentially life-threatening injuries, such as bleeding, to ensure you are not missing anything vital.

Loosen any tight clothing such as ties, scarves and belts.

Look to establish how an injury may have been caused. Look for clues, for example, are they on a road or is there a ladder beside them? If you suspect they've fallen from a height, been hit at speed or banged their head, a spinal injury is a possibility and although protecting the airway is a priority, keep them as still as possible and avoid twisting their spine.

Head and neck:

- Monitor their breathing. Are they having any difficulties? Is it unusually fast, slow, laboured or noisy?
- Check their pulse - strong, weak, regular, irregular, fast or slow?
- Look at the size of their pupils - are they equal, unequal, large or small?
- Check for any bruising or bleeding
- Look at clues as to how the accident happened, could they have injured their neck and have a spinal injury?

Shoulders and chest:

- Are the shoulders equal, any sign of a fracture?
- For a conscious casualty, can they take a deep breath? Does the chest move easily and equally on both sides? Does it cause pain?
- Look for any bleeding. If you think they may have been shot, there is likely to be one wound in and another out. For a stabbing, there may be substantial internal damage and bleeding.

Abdomen and pelvis:

- Be very careful - do **not** squeeze or rock the pelvis in case it is damaged.
- Gently touch their abdomen and check if it causes any pain or discomfort.

Legs and arms:

- Check for signs of deformity, bruising or other indications that they may have a broken bone.
- Ask a conscious casualty if they can move their arms and legs and feel you touching them.
- Look for any signs of a weakness down one side.

Pockets:

- Be very careful looking in someone's pockets. People may have needles, weapons or drugs in there. Ensure there is a reliable witness as otherwise people may suspect you of pick pocketing them.

- Look for any other clues such as needle marks, medic alert bracelets or pendants, medication etc.

Unconscious and not breathing

CPR – Cardio Pulmonary Resuscitation

When you are resuscitating someone, you are acting as a life support machine. By pushing on someone's chest you are doing the job of their heart and when you breathe into them you are doing the job of their lungs. You are keeping their heart and brain oxygenated (i.e. keeping them alive), so when a defibrillator is deployed there is a good chance of bringing them back to life.

If they are not breathing or there are less than 2 normal breaths in a 10 second period, start CPR and phone for an ambulance.

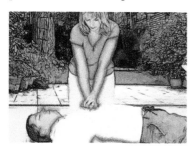

It is vital to resuscitate if you are unsure – much better to attempt to resuscitate someone who doesn't need it than fail to resuscitate someone who does.

When an adult or post-pubescent is unresponsive and not breathing, they are likely to still have oxygenated blood in their system. Their heart is no longer working effectively and it is therefore important to quickly circulate that oxygenated blood by pushing hard and fast on their chest.

- Kneel up so you are over the casualty
- Lock your elbows and push on the centre of their chest with the heel of your hands, one on top of the other
- Push down 5-6 cm (roughly a third of their chest)
- Do it at a rate of 115-120 beats per minute – roughly 2 per second
- Do 30 of these chest compressions then give 2 breaths

To give breaths:

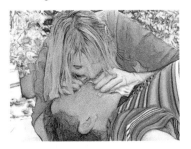

- **Tilt the head** and **lift the chin** to take the tongue off the back of the airway

- Hold their **nose**

- Give **2 breaths,** sealing your mouth around theirs and blowing into them like a balloon

If available, use a **face shield** to protect yourself.

Keep going – you are acting as a life support machine.

Do not expect them to regain consciousness without a defibrillator.

Make sure their chest rises each time. If it doesn't, try tilting the head a bit more.

If it still doesn't rise, go straight back to the compressions.

NOTE: If you are unable or unwilling to give an adult rescue breaths, just do chest compressions. This will give them an additional 3-4 minutes they won't have otherwise and is much better than not doing anything. Babies and children will always need breaths to give them the best chance.

If there is someone else to help, do cycles of 30 compressions and 2 breaths and swap every 2 minutes.

If you are on your own, call an ambulance as soon as you realise the casualty is unresponsive and not breathing.

Resuscitating a child (pre-puberty)

1. **Tilt the head** and **lift the chin** to take the tongue off the back of the airway.

2. Give **5 rescue breaths** to re-oxygenate them. *Children do not keep residual oxygen in their system as adults do, and a breathing problem is more likely to be the cause of their respiratory arrest (than a heart attack, for example).*

3. Making sure their head is tilted, hold their nose, seal your mouth round theirs and blow into them like a balloon.

4. Make sure their chest rises each time – if it doesn't, you may need to open the airway a little more.

5. Circulate the oxygenated blood by giving chest compressions, using the same technique as for adults but with only **one hand** on their chest.

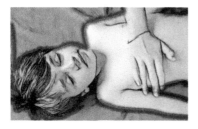

Push down by **1/3 of the depth** of their chest – ideally with one hand, otherwise use two to ensure you get the depth that you need.

Push at a rate of **120 beats per minute - about 2 per second.**

After the initial 5 breaths and 30 compressions, give them 2 more breaths and then continue with the compressions again. Alternate 30 compressions: 2 breaths (as with adults).

For a baby or child, if you are on your own, you should perform a minute's CPR before phoning 999 (5 breaths, 30:2, 30:2 is about a minute).

Resuscitating a Baby

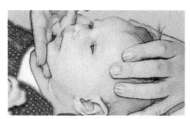

Carefully **tilt the head** and **lift the chin** to roughly a horizontal position to take the tongue off the back of the airway. **Give 5 rescue breaths** to re-oxygenate them.

Do **not** tilt a baby's head all the way back - just to horizontal.

Tilt the head and lift the chin

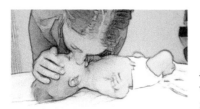

First check for **Danger, Response, Airway and Breathing.** If you are not sure whether they are breathing, or if they are not breathing normally, you will need to start **CPR.**

Give 5 rescue breaths

Seal your mouth around their mouth and nose if you can fit your mouth over both and blow into them gently with a puff of your cheeks. A baby's lungs are about the size of a tea bag, so don't blow too hard - just hard enough to inflate the chest.

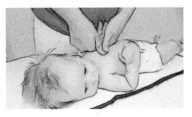

Make sure their chest rises each time. If it doesn't, you probably haven't opened the airway sufficiently. Re-adjust and try again.

You will then need to circulate the oxygenated blood by pushing down hard and fast on their chest with two fingers or your thumbs.

Push down 1/3 of the depth of the chest between the nipples

- Push hard and fast on the centre of their chest, roughly between the nipples.

- Push down by a third of the depth of their chest, pushing hard enough to get the depth you need.

Do this at a rate of 110-120 beats per minute - roughly 2 per second.

After the first 5 breaths and 30 compressions, give them 2 more short sharp breaths and then continue with the compressions again. **Alternate 30 compressions and 2 breaths.**

Keep going - You are being a life support machine and keeping them alive

If you are on your own, you should perform a minute's CPR before phoning for an ambulance (5 breaths, 30:2, 30:2 is about a minute)

If there is an AED machine, use it!

If you can share the CPR with someone, you should change every 2 minutes to prevent exhaustion. Do a couple of rotations each and have the minimum possible delay when changing over.

(Paediatric First Responders in a medical setting e.g. doctors and nurses in neonatal care and paediatric A&E are taught different numbers of breaths and compressions. The ratios specified in this course are those re commended by the Resuscitation Guidelines for lay responders.)

When to phone an ambulance

For a baby or child: If you are on your own, you should perform 1 minute's CPR before phoning for an ambulance (5 breaths, 30:2, 30:2 is about a minute).

For an adult, phone for an ambulance as soon as you realise that they are unresponsive and not breathing. Put the phone on the speaker option.

Hygiene during CPR

When someone is unconscious, everything is relaxed and the casualty is likely to passively vomit, which is unpleasant if you are in the process of doing mouth-to-mouth resuscitation. It is unlikely that you would catch anything serious from someone you were resuscitating, but you should use a face shield to protect yourself from any possible risk.

If you do not have a professional mask or face shield, use an improvised face shield e.g. a shirt, scarf or plastic bag with a hole in it. This will allow you to resuscitate without it being too intimate and unpleasant. However, it will not protect you from blood, vomit or infection.

- If they start to gurgle when you breathe into them, briefly roll them onto their side and empty as much vomit as possible from their mouth before continuing with the breaths. Otherwise you could be blowing vomit into their lungs.

Defibrillators/AEDs - what they are and how to use them

Hundreds of people are alive today entirely due to the prompt and appropriate use of a defibrillator. Automatic External Defibrillators (A EDs) ar e no w easily accessible at numerous locations - train and tube stations, shopping centres, dentists, GP practices, sports grounds and leisure centres, and they're available for the public to use. They can be semi-automatic (you still need to press the shock button when indicated) or fully automatic (the machine shocks automatically when a shock is advised).

Why are they important?

Numerous studies have shown that if someone has a cardiac arrest in the community with no defibrillator immediately available, there is only a 6% chance of them surviving, even if someone is performing great CPR on them. Defibrillators save lives. The faster you can use a defibrillator and get the casualty advanced medical care, the greater their chance of survival.

AED statistics
New England Journal of Medicine 2000 343: 1206 - 120

	Survival rate
Current UK survival rates without immediate access to an AED	6%
Casualty in a shockable rythm and shock delivered within 3 minutes	74%
Every additional minute's delay before shock given = 10% reduction in mortality	

Where to find an AED

AEDs are becoming widely accessible in the community as many public places are now equipped with one.

Public machines are for anyone to use in an emergency. They usually have an alarm function to alert support staff that it is being used and have instructions to access the machine.

This sign is the official signage to show that there is an AED available.

Chain of survival

The sooner you recognise there is a problem, get help on the way, start CPR and use a defibrillator, the better the outcome.

What if you get it wrong?

A defibrillator is for use on someone who is unconscious and not breathing. You are unable to shock someone with a defibrillator if they don't need it, so you can't do any harm.

The machine analyses the casualty's heart rhythm and will only allow a shock to be given if they are in a shockable rhythm. It is not possible to override this with an AED and if the machine tells you that a shock is not advised, you should continue to give CPR until the ambulance arrives.

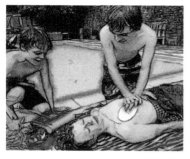

Ensure you know how to do the best CPR, pushing down 5-6 cm on the centre of the chest at a rate of about 2 compressions per second.

You cannot get it wrong with a defibrillator and you cannot make things worse!

The machine talks to you and tells you what to do.

The heart's electrical system

The heart is a unique organ in the body that is to generate its own electrical impulses and beat on its own even if the spinal cord has been severed.

All organs of the body require oxygenated blood to survive and the heart and lungs are key to making this happen. The heart pumps oxygenated blood through arteries around the body to provide the body's tissues with nutrients and oxygen. Veins bring blood back to the heart and lungs to be re-oxygenated and pumped back around the body again.

The heart is made up of 4 chambers - 2 smaller ones at the top (atria) that collect blood and squeeze it into the much larger pumping chambers (ventricles). The heart is prompted to contract and pump the blood around the body by electrical impulses.

The primary pacemaker (known as the sinoatrial node) initiates impulses that pass through the atria to make them contract.

The impulses stimulate the secondary pacemaker (atrioventricular node) which passes the impulse down the centre of the heart to the ventricles to cause them to contract from the bottom upwards expelling the blood out of the heart. The electrical cells then recharge ready to do it all over again. This is the basis of the ECG.

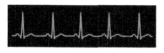

In sinus rhythm (the normal heart rhythm), the first bump represents the top chambers (atria) contracting, the peak is the ventricles contracting, and the final bump is the recharging of the impulse to do it again.

Ventricular fibrillation

If an area of heart muscle is damaged due to a heart attack, the casualty may well survive, depending on where the damage occurs and how much heart muscle is lost.

Because the heart has so many back-up systems, even if one of the pacemakers is damaged, the heart itself may still be able to generate sufficient electrical impulses to contract. The heart is an amazing organ comprising of cells capable of independently generating impulses and the 2 pacemakers work together and act like the conductor of an orchestra initiating the correct impulses and ensuring that the heart beats to a regular rhythm.

When an area of heart muscle is damaged, it becomes unstable and often fires off its own impulses independently; this interferes with the co-ordinated rhythm generated by the pacemakers.

This misfiring affects the rhythm of the heart and causes it to become irregular. If the heart experiences a 'misfiring' beat at the point when the cells are re-charging, this can upset the whole system and the different cells fire independently of each other causing the heart to quiver erratically and chaotically. This is known as ventricular fibrillation and while the heart is shaking instead of pumping, it is incapable of effectively circulating the blood around the body.

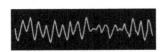
Ventricular fibrillation (VF) causes the casualty to become unconscious and stop breathing. VF is a shockable rhythm and if a defibrillator is used promptly on someone in VF, there is a strong chance that stopping the heart with the shock will allow the heart to restart in a normal rhythm. The longer someone remains in VF, the less likely it is that their heart will restart normally.

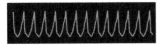
Ventricular tachycardia (VT) is another shockable rhythm. The heart rate has become so fast that the chambers are incapable of refilling and so there is little or no blood being pumped around the body. If the casualty is unconscious, a defibrillator will stop the heart and it may well start in a normal rhythm.

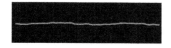 Asystole (flat-lining) - this is too late for an automated external defibrillator (AED), as the heart has run out of oxygen and is now still.

Using a defibrillator

A defibrillator does not jumpstart the heart like jumpstarting a car, it stops it, like rebooting a computer, allowing the individual heart cells to recharge simultaneously and the pacemaker in the heart to hopefully restart it in a normal rhythm.

Check for:

Danger – Do not put yourself in danger.

Response – If no response shout for help and if possible get a bystander to call for an ambulance and locate a defibrillator if there is one.

Airway – Open the airway and check for breathing.

Breathing – If the casualty does not appear to be breathing normally and there are less than 2 breaths in a 10 second period you will need to start CPR.

If you are on your own – Call 999/112 and get the AED as quickly as possible.

If you have help - Your bystander will need to let the emergency services know that the casualty is unconscious and not breathing and bring the AED as quickly as possible. Continue CPR while waiting for the defibrillator.

When the AED arrives

As soon as the AED arrives, it should be activated (usually done just by opening the lid, or pressing an obvious button). It will then start speaking to you. If there are 2 of you, one should continue with the CPR, while the other attaches the leads to the AED (if necessary), dries the chest (shaves them if excessively hairy) and places the pads on the chest as per the diagrams.

- Peel the pad off the backing one at a time and place onto the dry chest according to the diagram.
- Place one pad below the casualty's right collar bone.
- Place the other on the casualty's left hand side, over their lower ribs.

If you realise you have put the pads on the wrong way round, do not remove them as the AED will still work fine.

- The AED will analyse the heart rhythm. Stop CPR when instructed and ensure no one is touching the casualty.

If a shock is advised:

- Check the whole length of the casualty to ensure no one is touching them. Shout 'stand clear', loudly.
- Press the flashing shock button as directed (fully automated AEDs will do this automatically once a shock is advised).
- Continue with CPR as directed.
- Keep going with 30 compressions to 2 breaths.
- Do not stop to check them unless they begin to regain consciousness and start breathing normally.
- The machine will reassess their heart rhythm every 2 minutes and advise another shock if indicated.

If no shock is advised:

- Continue with CPR and follow prompts.
- Keep going until help arrives or the casualty begins to regain consciousness and starts to breathe normally.
- The machine will reassess their heart rhythm every 2 minutes and advise a shock if indicated.

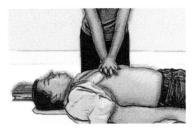
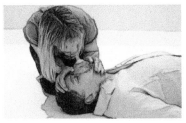

30 compressions   2 rescue breaths

If there is more than one rescuer, swap every couple of minutes.

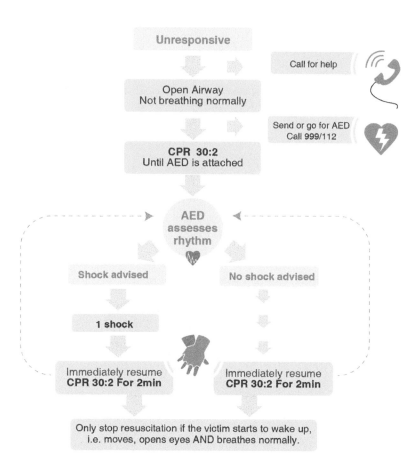

Things to keep with your defibrillator

- Spare pads and paediatric pads if required
- Resuscitation mask
- Tough-cut scissors to remove clothes
- Gloves
- Towel to dry the chest
- A razor to shave an excessively hairy chest

Safety considerations when using an AED

- Electric shock - The risk of electric shock from an AED is extremely small. Providing the chest is dry and the pads are well stuck, there is little chance of the charge arcing and causing a problem. However, it is always sensible to check no one is touching the casualty when the shock is given.

- Jewellery - Avoid placing the pads over metal jewellery as it can conduct electricity and burn the casualty. Jewellery does not need to be removed, just moved out of the way.

- Ensure the casualty is still when the AED is analysing the rhythm, to avoid an inappropriate rhythm assessment. Switch off vehicle engines and vibrating machinery if possible.

- Medication patches - Remove any obvious patches on the casualty's chest and do not place pads over them. Some heart patients wear GTN (glyceryl tri-nitrate) patches and these would explode if a shock was passed over them.

- Implanted devices - most pacemakers are on the left-hand side of the chest. Don't place pads over strange bumps or scars.

- Flammable atmosphere - turn off oxygen when giving the shock, do not use in the presence of petrol fumes.

Using a defibrillator on a child

Placement of paediatric pads

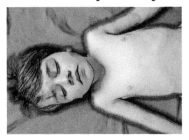

Paediatric pads are usually placed one on the front of the child's chest and one in the middle of their back.

Sometimes they are placed in the same location as adult pads - look at the diagram on the packet.

Some defibrillators have a switch or key that adapts it for child use. If you have a child over the age of 1 who needs a defibrillator, but only have adult pads available, adult pads can be used on the front of the child's chest and the other placed in the centre of their back as per the diagram above. If it is a baby that needs resuscitating, you must use paediatric pads or the paediatric capability.

AED signage

The Resuscitation Council has produced a standard sign to indicate the presence of an AED and this has been endorsed by the Health and Safety Executive. The sign is freely downloadable from the Resuscitation Council.

Maintenance of the AED

- Follow the manufacturer's recommendations for the maintenance of the AED.

- It should be kept in a prominent place and ideally everyone in the building should have easy access to it and know where it is kept.

- Check the expiry date for the battery and pads and order replacements in good time. Spare pads and a battery are highly recommended.

- Most AEDs have warning lights and alarms to alert you if there is a malfunction or if the battery is running low. Ideally, the AED should be briefly checked daily to ensure it is in good working order if you need it.

- Most units have a battery life of around 5 years.

When the paramedics arrive

The paramedics will need to know what happened, how long you have been doing CPR, whether a shock was advised by the AED and if so, how many shocks have been given.

After the emergency:

- Ensure that appropriate paperwork and accident forms are completed

- The British Heart Foundation and Association of Ambulance Medical Directors in partnership with the University of Warwick have a national out-of-hospital database of community cardiac arrests and would welcome your input:

    www2.warwick.ac.uk/fac/med/research/hscience/ctu/trials/other/ohcao/aed

- Restock anything that has been used

- Ensure that everyone is OK afterwards and make time to talk things through.
- It is perfectly normal to feel any of the following:
    - A feeling of elation and an adrenaline buzz
    - Anger
    - Confusion
    - Flashbacks and bad dreams
    - Depression

Dealing with a medical emergency can be extremely stressful and some people need professional help and counselling following such an episode.

PART 3

TREATMENT FOR COMMON INJURIES AND ILLNESSES

The third part of the book takes you through common medical emergencies.

We start with choking and breathing problems, then work through major and minor bleeds, burns, head injuries, broken bones, soft tissue injuries and many other possible childhood injuries and illnesses.

Choking

Choking occurs when something gets stuck in the back of the throat and blocks the airway. When it is partially blocked, the casualty can usually cough and still make noises. When it is totally blocked, the casualty is unable to make any sound at all. Choking can occur in any age group, but is more common with small children and the elderly.

Choking is frightening, both for the casualty and for the person trying to help. The calmer you can be while assisting, the calmer the casualty will be. Stress and panic make things worse.

How to help a choking adult or teenager

Choking is most often caused by people laughing or speaking while eating, swallowing food before it has been completely chewed or putting things such a pen tops in their mouths.

If you come across someone who's choking:

- Stay as calm as you can and try and keep everyone else calm too.

- Always check first to see if someone can cough and encourage them to do so. Often they are able to clear the blockage themselves.

- If they are coughing, let them cough.

- If they are not coughing, remind them to cough, as they may be able to clear the obstruction themselves.

If they are unable to cough:

Bend them forward supporting them on their chest with the other hand and use the heel of your hand to **give a sharp back blow** between the shoulder blades. Check to see if the blockage has cleared before giving another blow. If the blockage hasn't cleared after five blows, get someone to phone an ambulance and try abdominal thrusts/Heimlich manoeuvre:

- Stand behind them and place one hand in a fist under their rib cage. Use the other hand to pull up and under to dislodge the obstruction. You are using a J-shaped motion to pull up and under their rib cage. Perform abdominal thrusts **up to 5 times**, checking between each one if the obstruction has been cleared. Anyone who has received abdominal thrusts must be seen by a doctor.

- If the person is still choking, **call 999 (or 112)** if you haven't already, and alternate five back blows and five abdominal thrusts until emergency help arrives. **If at any point the person becomes unconscious, commence CPR.**

What to do when a child is choking

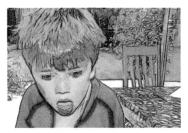

Babies and young children can choke on anything that can fit through a loo roll. To prevent choking: keep small objects out of reach, cut up food into very small pieces and supervise children while they're eating, especially if they're under five years old.

If a child shows signs of choking, stay calm and ask them to cough to help remove the object. If this doesn't work, follow the steps below to clear a blockage.

Signs of choking:

- Unable to speak or cry

- Clutching their throat

- Struggling to breathe

-

What to do

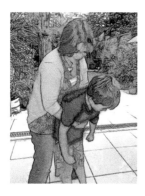

- Bend the child forward, supporting them on their chest with the other hand.

- Use the flat of your hand to give a firm back blow between the shoulder blades.

- Check to see if the blockage has cleared before giving another blow.

If the back blows haven't helped, get an ambulance on the way.

If the blockage hasn't cleared after five blows, try abdominal thrusts/the Heimlich manoeuvre:

- Stand behind the child and place one hand in a fist between their tummy button and their rib cage. Use the other hand to pull up and under in a J-shaped motion, to dislodge the obstruction. Perform abdominal thrusts up to 5 times, checking each time to see if the obstruction has cleared. Anyone who has received abdominal thrusts must be seen by a doctor.

If the child is still choking, **call 999 (or 112)** if you haven't already and alternate five back blows and five abdominal thrusts until emergency help arrives. If at any point the child becomes unconscious, commence **CPR.**

What to do when a baby is choking

Clearing a blockage - babies under 1 year

* First look in the baby's mouth and if there is something obvious in the mouth, remove it with finger tips.

DO NOT put your fingers down a baby or child's throat, or finger sweep the mouth, as this can make matters worse by pushing the obstruction further down or by causing swelling.

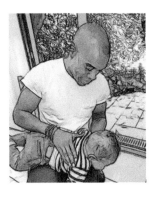

* Lay the baby downwards on your forearm or across your legs, supporting them under their chin and using the flat of your hand, give **a firm back blow between the shoulder blades.**

* Give up to five back blows and check between each blow to see if the blockage has cleared. **If they are still choking, call the emergency services and start chest thrusts straight away.**

* If the obstruction hasn't cleared, put the baby on their back, place two fingers in the centre of the chest just below the nipple line and give up to five chest thrusts.

Warning: never do abdominal thrusts on a baby under a year as you could cause damage. Use chest thrusts instead.

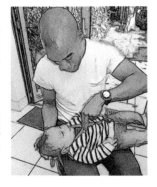

* Check to see if the blockage has cleared between each chest thrust.

* If the baby is still choking, call 999/112, if you haven't already, and continue to alternate five back blows and five chest thrusts until emergency help arrives.

Unresponsive and not breathing	
Adult (post puberty)	**Child or baby**
999/112	5 Rescue breaths first
Start CPR!	Start CPR!
30 compression: 2 breaths	30 compressions: 2 breaths **On your own with a child?** **CPR for 1 minute, then 999/112**

If the obstruction comes out:

If they are unconscious but breathing, put them in the recovery position.

If they are unconscious and not breathing, start CPR.

If they seem fine, ensure they don't have problems swallowing and check there is no pain or bleeding. It is always advisable to have them checked out by a medical professional. If it is not your child, ensure you have contacted their parents.

If the child has been given abdominal thrusts or chest thrusts, they should always be checked by a medical professional.

Drowning

Always ensure basic safety around water. Children should always be supervised as they can drown in surprisingly small amounts of water. They should never be left alone in a bath, even for a short time. Be vigilant around pools and ponds which should have safety features, such as fencing and gates. Drowning can happen quickly and quietly (unlike the way it is portrayed in films) and causes a frightening number of fatalities every year.

Generally, drowning casualties do not inhale large amounts of water. Most deaths from drowning are caused from secondary drowning (see below), or from a muscle spasm in the throat that causes the airway to block.

However, drowning casualties do tend to swallow large amounts of water and are thus very likely to vomit. When resuscitating, you should be aware of this and that you may need to turn them onto their side periodically to ensure that they do not inhale vomit into their lungs.

NOTE: for lifeguards and those trained in water rescue, if you have been trained to give rescue breaths before compressions, continue with this protocol.

If you are aware that someone is drowning:

1. If they are unconscious in water, remove them from it as quickly as you can, but **never put yourself in danger**. Do not enter the water to rescue a drowning casualty unless you have been trained to do so. Throw a lifebelt or rope if possible, otherwise get help fast.

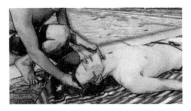

2. As soon as you get onto dry land, turn them on their back, tilt the head and lift the chin to clear the airway. If there is a defibrillator available, you should use it immediately.

3. Check for breathing and if there isn't any, start resuscitation immediately.

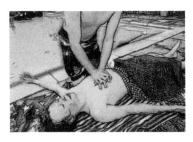

4. If it is an adult, start with 30 chest compressions pushing down hard and fast followed by 2 rescue breaths. For a child or baby, start with 5 rescue breaths then alternate 30 compressions and 2 breaths, as with adults. If at any point you are aware of vomit, briefly turn them onto their side to remove it and then roll them onto their back again to resume resuscitation.

5. If it is warm and they haven't been in the water very long, you may find they start to regain consciousness quickly. If this happens, swiftly put them into the recovery position to help them drain water and vomit. Keepchecking they're still breathing.

6. If it is cold, they will not start to regain consciousness until their body is warm enough

7. Do 30 compressions to 2 breaths and keep going - grab a coat or something to put over them.

8. Call for the emergency services and keep going.

If you are a qualified lifeguard, you will have been taught to give 5 rescue breaths first whether you are rescuing an adult or child – this is a specific modification to the training for lifeguards.

IMPORTANT: secondary drowning

Anyone who has been unconscious in the water should be assessed in hospital, as there is a real risk of suffering secondary drowning. Secondary drowning can occur due to even a small amount of water entering the lungs. The lungs become inflamed and irritated and start drawing fluid from the blood supplying the lungs into the alveoli (the air pockets of the lungs).

This reaction can happen up to 72 hours after the casualty has appeared to have recovered and is life-threatening. The casualty may deteriorate suddenly and develop severe difficulty breathing. If this happens, phone an ambulance immediately.

Asthma

Asthma is a common condition in which airways go into spasm and cause tightness of the chest and severe difficulty breathing when someone is exposed to something that irritates their airways. The airways become narrow, then their lining becomes inflamed and can start producing sticky mucus or phlegm which makes it hard to breathe.

Asthma can occur in people of all ages. If the symptoms are well controlled, it should not rule out any form of physical activity. Often symptoms become harder to control at certain times of the year or in particular weather conditions. An asthmatic should remain vigilant and ensure they have sufficient in-date reliever inhaler medication with them at all times.

What causes asthma

If there is a family history of asthma, eczema or allergies, you are more likely to develop asthma. Research has also shown that smoking during pregnancy significantly increases the risk of a child developing asthma. Similarly, children whose parents smoke are more likely to develop asthma.

Note: Asthma UK has a great programme to help children with asthma and their parents and carers to manage their asthma and live a full and active life.

People with asthma should always have their **blue reliever inhaler** quickly accessible.

Asthma can be triggered by all sorts of things:

- Exercise can trigger attacks. However, people should not avoid exercise because they are asthmatic - they should always have their blue reliever inhaler with them.

- Chemicals.

- Smoke and fumes.

- Cold air.

- Colds and viruses.

- Stress.

- Household dust, fungi, moulds and pollen.

- Some people have specific allergic triggers which bring on a major asthma attack in response to their specific allergens.

Asthma sufferers will learn what triggers their breathing problems.

Symptoms of asthma

- Coughing

- Wheezing

- Shortness of breath

- Tightness in the chest

- Often people find it particularly difficult to breathe out and have an increase in sticky mucus and phlegm

Not everyone will get all these symptoms. Some people experience them from time to time; a few may have them all the time.

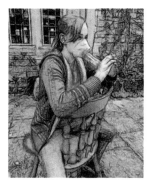

NOTE: Encouraging someone to sit upright may be helpful when dealing with breathing problems. Sitting the wrong way round on a chair may help.

DO NOT take them outside for fresh air if it is cold, as cold air can make symptoms worse.

Spacers

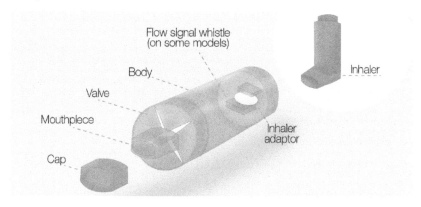

Using a spacer device has been shown to deliver the medication more effectively, minimising the amount not reaching the airways and just hitting the back of the throat. This gives people greater control of their asthma.

There are a huge variety of shapes and sizes, but not all spacers fit all types of inhalers - use the spacer prescribed with the inhaler. Spacers for smaller children are usually fitted with a face mask.

There is considerable co-ordination required to use an inhaler without a spacer and this can lead to increased stress and worsening of symptoms. Always keep the spacer with the inhaler and have both accessible at all times.

How to help in an asthma attack

The following guidelines are suitable for both children and adults:

- Be calm and reassuring as reducing stress and keeping the casualty calm helps them control their symptoms. Panic can increase the severity of an attack.

- Encourage the casualty to take one to two puffs of the reliever inhaler (usually blue). Use a spacer device if available.

- Sit them down, loosen any tight clothing and encourage them to take slow, steady breaths.

- If they do not start to feel better, they should take more puffs of their reliever inhaler. Do 2 every 2 minutes up to a maximum of 10 - or as prescribed.

- If they do not start to feel better after using the inhaler as above, or if you are worried at any time, call 999.

- Keep using the reliever inhaler while waiting for the paramedics.

People may have a variety of different asthma inhalers and medication to control their asthma; if they are having an asthma attack it is the reliever inhaler that they need.

After an emergency asthma attack, the casualty should make an appointment with a doctor or asthma nurse for an asthma review. This should be within 48 hours of their attack.

Croup

Croup is a common childhood infection of the upper airways, where the larynx and the trachea become infected and swollen. It occurs most often in children from 3 months to 5 years, often during autumn or winter. Children are typically unwell with cold-like symptoms, a slightly raised temperature, are wheezy, with a cough that sounds like a sea-lion barking. The infection is caused by a virus and so antibiotics will not help. Symptoms are often a lot worse at night. Humidifying a room used to be recommended, but it has been shown that this can spread the infection to other areas such as the epiglottis, which can be more dangerous.

If your baby gets much worse in the night and you are concerned, phone for an ambulance and they will bring nebulisers to ease their breathing. Croup is not life-threatening, but epiglottis has similar symptoms and is serious.

Croup is characterised by rapid shallow breathing, a barking cough and a highpitched wheezy noise when the child breathes in.

- Taking your child outside on a mild evening can ease symptoms, however taking them out if it is very cold can make things worse.

- If the child's breathing becomes very wheezy and laboured, their lips start to appear blue or they are getting worse, phone for an ambulance immediately.

- Usually it is a mild illness, but can be very scary if they appear to be struggling to breathe. If you are at all worried, seek medical help.

- If the child is unwell and having difficulty breathing, it is important that you remain calm as additional stress and panic will make their symptoms worse.

- As it is a breathing problem, they are likely to be more comfortable in an upright position.

- Paediatric paracetamol can be helpful in reducing their fever and makingthem more comfortable.

Never give cough medication for croup as it can make a child drowsy and is unlikely to be effective. Never put your fingers down their throat as this can cause their throat muscles to spasm and block their airway.

Panic attacks and hyperventilation

Most people have experienced a sense of panic at some time in their life and this is a perfectly normal reaction. Panic is an extreme feeling of fear and dread and the overwhelming desire to escape an uncomfortable situation. Panic attacks can be when these feelings become extreme, or can happen for no apparent reason.

The physical feelings may be frightening and can include the following:

- A pounding and racing heart, even palpitations (feeling your heart is stopping or missing beats).

- Shortness of breath or a feeling of choking.

- Shaking, tingling or numbness in your fingers and toes.

- Feeling sick, dizzy, sweating and needing the loo.

- Thinking you might die.

- Feeling you are losing control of your mind or that you are going crazy.

- An aggressive desire to escape.

Difficulty breathing due to panic attacks should not be confused with asthma. Asthma can be life-threatening. The casualty needs their medication and help quickly, whereas panic attacks are usually short-lived and the casualty will make a full recovery.

During an asthma attack the person is often wheezy as they are struggling to breathe, whereas large volumes of air can be heard entering and leaving the lungs of a hyperventilating casualty.

- Reassure them calmly and clearly. They may not be able to explain what has caused them to panic, so do not pressure them to do this. Your supportive presence should help.

- Speak to them in positive terms - "you will be okay, this will pass in a minute" etc.

- Remove them from anything obvious causing distress.

- Encourage them to breathe calmly and slowly, in and out through their nose to reduce the amount of carbon dioxide being lost.

- Small sips of water may help to calm them.

- If symptoms get worse, get medical help.

- When the panic attack is over, talk it through with them, and speak to their parents, teachers or friends, with their consent. Discuss relaxation techniques and other helpful means of coping if this happens again.

Do not suggest breathing in and out of a paper bag. People used to suggest that breathing in and out of a paper bag was helpful during a panic attack. The physiology makes sense, as breathing out in a panic will result in a loss of carbon dioxide in the blood, and breathing into a bag will restore the lost CO_2 and build up the levels again.

However, the danger with a paper bag is that the casualty becomes dependent upon it and can panic if they do not have one to hand. It is also dangerous for someone having an asthma attack to be encouraged to do this and may make things substantially worse.

If the attacks are persistent and severe, the casualty can be referred for specialist help.

Anaphylactic shock

What is an allergic reaction?

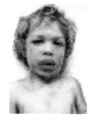

Allergic reactions occur because the body's immune system reacts inappropriately in response to the presence of a substance that it wrongly perceives as a threat. In order to develop an allergic response, the body has to be exposed to something to trigger the immune response - this can be touched, inhaled, swallowed or injected - during a routine vaccination or by an insect sting.

Picture thanks to the
Anaphylaxis Campaign

The body doesn't react to the irritant directly, but reacts to the histamine released by cells damaged through the immune response on subsequent exposure.

What causes an allergic reaction?

Everyone makes antibodies, but people prone to allergic reactions produce more than most. When someone with an allergic predisposition is exposed to an allergen, they produce a lot of antibodies that bind to the mast cells in the tissues.

When the antibodies line up next to each other, the reaction affects the membrane and causes the cell to break down. The breaking down of these cells releases histamine and other chemicals.

Anaphylactic reaction

This mechanism is so sensitive that minute quantities of the allergen can cause a reaction. The released chemicals act on blood vessels to cause the swelling in the mouth and anywhere on the skin. In asthmatics, the effect may be mainly on the lungs, causing a severe asthma attack for which an inhaler is no help.

Antihistamine can be effective for minor reactions

We all normally have small amounts of histamine in our system and it is important for various vital functions of the body including regulating stomach acid and as a neurotransmitter in our nerve cells. However, larger amounts of histamine being released leads to symptoms such as sneezing, blocked nose, itching… the sort of symptoms often associated with hay fever and mild allergies. Antihistamine medication can work effectively at resolving these symptoms. However, it is important to note that antihistamine medication typically takes around 15 minutes to work.

Anaphylaxis is life threatening

Life threatening and systemic allergic reactions are caused by the body producing even more histamine, which dilates small blood vessels and causes them to leak, resulting in swelling in areas such as the lungs - leading to breathing problems. Sufferers may have a rash and be flushed due to the increased blood supply to the skin. Their blood pressure could drop dramatically and they may collapse.

The more times someone is exposed to the substance they react to, the quicker and more severe the reaction may be.

If they don't have a rash associated with the symptoms, it could still be an anaphylactic reaction. If they have a rapid onset of symptoms and may have been exposed to an allergen, treat it as an anaphylactic reaction.

Who is at greatest risk from anaphylaxis?

It is thought that people can inherit the predisposition to react to a specific allergen, combined with environmental factors. People can develop reactions to things that have never previously been a problem. If there is a family history, there is a far greater chance of someone having allergic tendencies.

If a patient has suffered a bad allergic reaction in the past - whatever the cause, this may make them more prone to having further severe reactions. If a significant reaction to a tiny dose occurs, or a reaction has occurred with just skin contact, this could indicate that they are sensitive to this specific allergen and greater contact could lead to a more severe attack.

Asthma can put a patient in a higher risk category. Most schools have at least one child at risk of acute allergic reaction. It is crucial that anyone caring for a child or working with someone with a history of anaphylaxis has detailed medical information about them and precisely what they are allergic to and what other products or foodstuffs may contain these allergens. Allergens can be contained in some obscure products that you wouldn't automatically associate them with, so if someone appears to be having a reaction, with no obvious trigger, use their adrenaline auto-injector if indicated and get emergency help quickly.

Teachers should think of all aspects of the school environment and ensure that children are not exposed to triggers when doing craft, junk modelling, cookery and all other aspects of the curriculum.

Common triggers for reactions

Food triggers

- The most common food triggers are: peanuts, tree nuts (e.g. almonds, walnuts, cashews, and Brazil nuts), sesame, fish, shellfish, dairy products and eggs.

Non-food triggers

- Non-food causes include wasp or bee stings, natural latex (rubber), penicillin or any other drug or injection.
- Exercise can also trigger a delayed allergic reaction following exposure to an allergen.

How to recognise an acute allergic reaction?

Common symptoms include:

- Generalised flushing of the skin.

- A rash or hives anywhere on the body.

- A feeling of anxiety or 'sense of impending doom'.

- Swelling of throat and mouth and difficulty in swallowing or speaking.

- Alterations in heart rate - usually a speeding up of the heart.

- Severe asthma attack which isn't relieved by an inhaler.

- Acute abdominal pain, violent nausea and vomiting.

- A sudden feeling of weakness followed by collapse and unconsciousness.

A patient is unlikely to experience all of the above symptoms.

How to Treat anaphylaxis

- The key advice is to avoid any known allergens if possible.

- If someone is having a mild allergic reaction, an antihistamine tablet or syrup can be very effective. However, the medication will take at least 15 minutes to work. If you are concerned that the reaction could be systemic (all over) and life-threatening, use an adrenaline auto-injector immediately. It is far better to give adrenaline and not to have needed it, than to have left it too late.

- Adrenaline auto-injectors are prescribed for those believed to be at risk.

- Adrenaline (also known as epinephrine) acts quickly to constrict blood vessels, relax smooth muscles in the lungs to improve breathing, stimulate the heartbeat and help to stop swelling around the face and lips.

- Acute allergic reactions can be life threatening and it is crucially important that you recognise the problem and know what to do quickly to save someone's life.

- Adrenaline works best if it is given as soon as you recognise that someone is having a reaction. You should administer the injector, or help the sufferer to administer it themselves, as quickly as possible and call for an ambulance stating clearly that the person is having an acute anaphylactic reaction.

- Adrenaline should rapidly treat all of the most dangerous symptoms of anaphylaxis, including throat swelling, difficulty breathing, and low blood pressure. However, the sufferer is likely to need additional medication in hospital to control the reaction.

- Adrenaline is metabolised very quickly - it is very important that you call an ambulance as soon as an auto-injector has been given as its effects can wear off within about 15 minutes. Another injector can be given 5-15 minutes after the first if necessary.

- **Phone for an ambulance immediately**

How to use an adrenaline auto-injector

Types of auto-injectors most commonly found in the UK::

How to use an Epipen

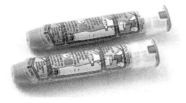

Auto-injectors

There are currently 3 common makes of adrenaline auto-injectors on the market in the UK: Epipen, Jext and Emerade. They all contain adrenaline and are all given in a similar manner. Epipen is the most popular in the UK.

Carry it with you at all times

If you are prescribed an adrenaline auto-injector you should always carry it with you and register to receive a reminder when it is going out of date. If you have been prescribed 2 adrenaline injectors as a duo pack, you should always carry both with you in case a second dose is needed. Teach friends and family what to do if they need to help you or someone else having an anaphylactic reaction.

Videos showing how to use adrenaline auto-injector are available on the drug company websites.

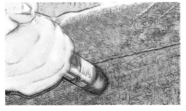

Hold the injector in your dominant hand and with the other hand, remove the safety cap. Put the injector firmly into the upper outer part of the casualty's thigh and hold it there for 10 seconds. Remove it carefully and they should begin to feel better quite quickly. If they continue to get worse, you may need to give another injector. The auto-injector can be given through clothes.

Always phone an ambulance.

Patient positioning for anaphylaxis

Someone suffering from acute anaphylaxis is also likely to be showing signs of clinical shock.

Reassuring the casualty, positioning them appropriately and keeping them warm and dry can make a major difference to their recovery.

Position someone suffering from anaphylactic shock, taking account of their symptoms, as follows:

If they are short of breath

If someone is very short of breath, they should be encouraged to sit in an upright position to help their breathing. Put something under their knees to help increase their circulation. This is the lazy W position.

If they are not short of breath, but are feeling lightheaded and dizzy

If they are not having difficulty breathing, but are feeling sick, dizzy and showing the signs and symptoms of shock, they should lie down with their legs raised to help increase the circulation to their vital organs. Encourage them to turn their head to one side if they are likely to vomit. They should be covered to keep them warm and kept in this position until the paramedics arrive.

Do not get them up until they have been medically assessed.

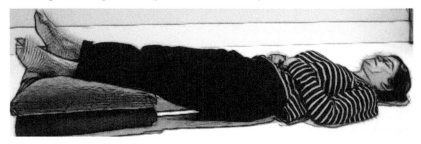

Treat for shock if they are showing symptoms of shock and are not having breathing problems.

After an anaphylactic reaction

An ambulance should always be called if someone is showing the signs of anaphylaxis and they will usually be admitted overnight for observation. This is because some people have a second reaction some hours after the first.

Don't forget to replace the used adrenaline auto-injector.

Wounds and bleeding

How to treat a bleeding wound

WEAR GLOVES WHEN DEALING WITH BLEEDING

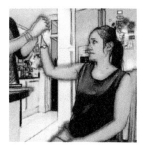 Always dispose of soiled dressings in a yellow incinerator bag, or in a sanitary bin.

- If someone is bleeding, the priority is to stop the blood coming out! This is completely logical except when someone is near a sink, as people automatically want to wash their wound under the tap, losing their precious blood in the process!

- The injury will be cleaned in hospital if they need medical attention or can be cleaned later (after you have given immediate first aid) if you are dressing it yourself.

- Encourage the casualty to sit or lie down in the most appropriate position for the location of the wound and the amount of blood lost - if they are feeling dizzy and showing early signs of shock, raise their legs.

- Put on your gloves and examine the wound to quickly assess:

    - The type and extent of bleeding

    - The source of the bleeding

    - Whether there are any foreign objects embedded in the wound - if so, do not remove them as they will be stemming the bleeding, but apply direct pressure either side of the object.

- Apply direct pressure to try and control bleeding - if the bleeding is controlled with this direct pressure, keep holding for 10 minutes as it takes this amount of time for clots to form.

- Once bleeding is controlled, dress the wound - if the wound bleeds through the first dressing, apply another on top. If the wound bleeds through the second dressing, you should re-assess to ensure you are applying direct pressure to the source of the bleeding. If there is major blood loss and you are unable to control this with pressure, you should consider alternative options to stop the bleeding such as packing the wound or applying a tourniquet, if you have been trained to do so.

- Keep the casualty warm and dry and get emergency help fast.

Treatment for bleeding:

- **S**it or lie them down

- **E**xamine the wound

- **A**pply direct pressure

- **D**ress the wound

What if direct pressure will not stop bleeding?

If the person is pale, cold, clammy (cold sweat) and showing signs of shock, or if there is a lot of blood - help their circulation by lying them down and raising their legs whilst applying direct pressure to control the bleeding.

The majority of bleeding can be controlled by direct pressure and this is likely to be the first and only solution you need. However, if the bleeding is severe and pulsating from the wound, and you are unable to stop the blood loss, you should consider using a tourniquet or packing the wound to apply pressure directly to the source of the bleed.

Please note: Tourniquets and haemostatic dressings have been introduced as additional options to treat severe catastrophic bleeding; however, direct pressure remains the main choice of treatment and it will control bleeding in the majority of cases. The European Research Council 2015 guidelines state that haemostatic dressings and tourniquets should be used when direct pressure is either not possible or not effective.

In environments where a catastrophic bleed is likely, tourniquets and haemostatic dressings should be an integral part of the first aid kit and all first aiders should be trained in their use. More information on this can be found on www.firstaidforlife.org.uk/

Types of wounds and minor injuries

Grazes

Grazes are superficial injuries caused by some of the skin being scraped off to reveal a dirty wound. It is never a priority to clean the wound immediately, usually it can be patched up with a plaster and then a short time later, cleaned properly, when in an environment where you can wash your hands, wear gloves and use gauze and water, or sterile wipes to clean it thoroughly.

How to treat a graze

- Clean most of the dirt from around the wound with a cloth.

- Using sterile gauze and clean water, or a sterile wipe, clean from the inside of the wound outwards in one sweep.

- Throw away the gauze and using a new sterile piece, again wipe from the inside of the wound outwards. Discard the gauze and use another piece until the wound is completely clean and devoid of any dirt or grit.

- Irrigating the wound with clean water can be helpful, but stubborn dirt and grit will need to be removed with proper cleaning.

- Apply a non-adherent dressing pad, shiny side down onto the wound and secure with some tape or a dressing with a bandage.

The dressing can be removed at night to allow the air to get to the wound. Avoid soaking in a bath, or going swimming until the wound has healed properly.

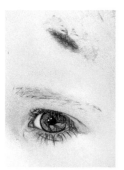

Any soiled dressings or gauze should be disposed of in an incinerator bin – either given to the emergency services to dispose of, or put into a sanitary bin. The casualty should also be encouraged to check their tetanus status.

Incised wound

A clean edged wound created by a sharp object.

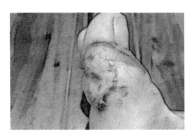

Laceration

This sort of wound involves a lot of tissue damage and often involves crushing and ripping of the body. It can look very frightening but the treatment is the same as for any other wound.

Puncture wound

Maybe caused by a sharp object with a deep track of internal damage, contamination and germs. There may b e a s mall e ntry wound t hat may h ave caused a lot of internal damage. A stab wound can be a type of puncture wound. Never remove an object left in the wound.

Contusion

This is another word for a bruise, which is bleeding under the skin. Apply a wrapped ice pack for 10 minutes to reduce bruising.

Knocked out teeth

A whole tooth that has been knocked out can be kept alive and re-implanted. Lost teeth can result from any severe hit in the mouth. It is particularly common with something like a swing hitting someone in the face, a cyclist being hit as a car door is opened or from fight.

Stop the bleeding

If someone is hit in the face and their tooth is knocked out complete with its root, you should advise the person to bite on a clean cloth to stem the bleeding.

Heads and faces bleed profusely as they have a good blood supply. Apply a wrapped ice pack to reduce the swelling to the face. Pick up the tooth (avoid touching the root) and it can be kept alive in milk or saliva. Transport the casualty and their tooth to a good dentist or a dental hospital and the tooth may be able to be re-implanted.

Wear gloves when dealing with bleeding.

Amputated parts

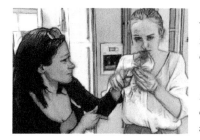

Amputated tips of fingers and toes are very common injuries and with the right initial first aid treatment, they can very often be successfully reattached.

Anything with a hinge can potentially remove a finger or toe. Be particularly careful with doors slamming, bicycle chains and anything sharp.

When part of the finger or toe is amputated

If part of a finger is amputated, the priority is to look after the casualty.

- Sit them down, reassure them and grab a cloth to apply direct pressure to the stump.

- Elevate the injured hand above the level of the heart. Do not worry about the amputated part until bleeding has been controlled and the casualty is calmer.

Save the amputated part

- Pick up the finger. Do not wash it.

- Wrap it in a cloth, put this in a plastic bag and then put on an ice pack.

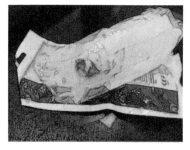

- Do not let the ice come directly into contact with the amputated part as it will cause ice burns and mean that the finger will not be able to be sewn back. You are chilling, not freezing the amputated part to prevent it decomposing. Transport the casualty and amputated finger to hospital, if necessary by ambulance.

Partially attached

If the finger is still partly attached with a blood supply, bandage the severed part carefully in situ. Support and elevate the hand and get emergency medical help.

Crushed and bruised fingers

If fingers are crushed and bruised, but no bits are missing, run the injured area under cool running water for 10 minutes, then apply a wrapped ice pack. Elevate the injured hand and seek medical advice.

Eye injuries

Eye injuries can be very unpleasant and painful. If someone has grit or dust in their eye that is moving about freely, rinse it out with water.

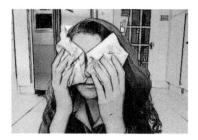

Something embedded in eye

If something is embedded in the eye, encourage the casualty to cover both eyes as moving one eye will result in the other eye moving. Never attempt to remove anything embedded in the eye.

Cuts to the eyelid

If someone has a cut to their eyelid, do not apply pressure. The best thing to do is to get a clean compress and then cover the eye with a small paper cup to prevent bacteria or debris from getting into the cut. Get medical help too.

Chemicals in the eye

If someone gets chemicals in their eye, wash the eye immediately with cold water or a saline eye wash and transport the person to the hospital.

- Wear gloves.
- Rinse the casualty's eye with cool running water for at least 10 minutes.
- Cover the affected eye with a non-fluffy pad if necessary.
- If you go to hospital, take details of the chemicals with you. If the chemicals have made the person sensitive to light, then cover their head with atowel before taking them to the hospital.

Nose bleeds

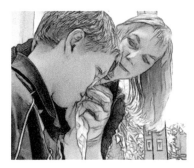

Small children frequently get nose bleeds as they have tiny blood vessels in their noses which dilate and burst when they get warm. Children often pick and poke their noses and are prone to running into things, all of which can result in bleeding noses. Weight lifters and people undertaking jobs that increase the blood pressure to their head are also prone to nose bleeds, as are elderly people with high blood pressure.

If someone has a nose bleed:

- Encourage them to sit down.

- Grab something to catch the blood.

- Lean the casualty forward, pinching the bridge of the nose. Leaning themforward whilst applying pressure to the nose will allow you to see when the bleeding has stopped and will avoid the blood trickling down the back of their throat which could make them sick.

- You should apply pressure externally on the nose to try and push the leaking blood vessel against the inside of the nose to compress it and stop it bleeding.

- Keep changing your grip until you have got to a point where no blood is coming out.

- Keep applying pressure for at least 10 minutes.

- Release pressure slightly and if it starts to bleed again, hold for another 10 minutes and then a further 10 minutes if necessary.

- Advise them not to pick, poke or blow the nose. If it starts again, you/they will need to apply pressure once again.

If it won't stop

If it really won't stop bleeding, you may need medical help.

Special situation

If the nose bleed has been caused by trauma, or a punch in the face, you may not be able to stop the bleeding. You need to apply pressure and try and reduce the amount of blood coming out, as loss of blood is dangerous. Apply a wrapped ice pack, keep applying pressure and get medical help.

Objects in nose

If a child puts an object up their nose, don't make a fuss and don't ask them to blow, as chances are, they are far more likely to sniff!

Take them down to A&E or to your doctor or nurse and ask them to remove it. It is not a medical emergency and so there is no immediate hurry, but it does need to be removed by a medical professional.

Objects in ears

If a child puts something in their ears, it is best for a medical professional to try and remove it. Don't try and fish it out yourself. The one exception is that if a nonstinging insect flies into their ear, pouring a small amount of water into the ear, may allow the fly to float out and save a trip to A&E. This is something for parents to do with their own children, it is not for child carers, as it is an invasive procedure.

Dressings

A dressing should be made of non-adherent material that will not stick to the wound. It should be sterile and just large enough to cover the wound completely.

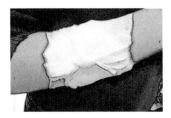

Applying a dressing

When applying a dressing, place the pad over the wound and firmly, but not too tightly, bandage over the top.

Check that you have not put it on too tightly by squeezing the nail bed of the finger – the colour should come back immediately when you let go.

If blood comes through the first dressing, put another on top in the same way. If it comes through both, apply direct pressure with another cloth, elevate and get medical help immediately. Be ready to treat for shock.

The purpose of a dressing

- Control bleeding
- Reduce the risk of shock
- Minimize the risk of infection, both to the first aider and to the casualty

Embedded objects

Do not remove the embedded object from the wound, as it will have damaged on the way in and will damage again on the way out! It may also be stemming any bleeding.

Apply pressure without pushing on the embedded object

- Use a rolled cloth or triangular bandage to make a donut ring and then apply pressure over the wound without pushing the object further in. Get medical help.

Either use 2 rolled bandages either side of the embedded object or a triangular bandage rolled into a donut ring.

- If you suspect that there is a glass in the wound, the casualty will need an x-ray.

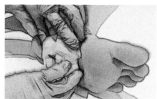

- Except for a small splinter that is clearly visible and easy to remove, nothing else should be removed from a wound. If the splinter is on a joint it should only be removed by a medical professional as it is possible that the joint capsule may have been damaged and this could lead to infection.

Removing a splinter

- Clean the wound with warm soapy water.
- Use a pair of clean tweezers, grip the splinter close to the skin and gently pull the splinter out at the same angle as it appears to have entered.

- Gently squeeze around the wound to encourage a little bleeding and ensure that there is nothing else remaining in the wound. Clean the wound once more and then cover with a breathable sterile dressing.

- Ensure the casualty's tetanus is up to date.

How much blood can you afford to lose?

Children have far less blood than adults. A person has approximately 0.5 litres of blood per 7kg of body weight or one pint of blood per stone (although this does not increase if someone is overweight). An 'average' adult has roughly 10 pints/6 litres of blood - at 40% blood loss the body can no longer compensate by constricting the blood vessels and making the heart pump faster. In a very major bleed, this could be as fast as 3-4 minutes.

The loss of a tea cup full of blood could be fatal for a baby, but please note that head and facial injuries often lose a lot of blood and can appear more frightening than they are: a cup full of blood would make a major mess!

The effect of blood loss for an average weight adult

Up to 0.5 litres:

Little or no effect on the body – equivalent to blood donation.

Up to 2 litres:
Adrenaline will be released which will speed up the pulse and cause sweating. The body starts to show the signs of shock.

More than 2 litres:
The pulse in the wrist can be undetectable as the body shuts down. Losing more blood will result in the casualty losing consciousness and the heart and breathing will eventually stop.

Shock

Shock is a lack of oxygen to the tissues of the body, usually caused by a fall in blood volume or blood pressure. Shock occurs when the body's circulatory system fails to work properly, which means that the tissues and organs of the body, including the heart and the brain, struggle to get sufficient oxygen. The body's response to this is to shut down the circulation to the skin - this causes the casualty to become pale, cold and clammy (cold, wet skin). The heart speeds up as it tries to get sufficient blood supply and oxygen around the body and blood supply is drawn away from the gut to prioritise vital organs - this causes the casualty to feel sick and thirsty. They may also feel anxious, dizzy and a bit confused as their brain suffers from the lack of oxygenated blood. If shock is untreated it can be fatal.

Shock results from major drop in blood pressure and is serious; it should not be confused with the frightened reaction people have when faced with a scary situation. It is clinical shock that often results in people dying from an acute injury or illness.

The most common types of shock are:

Hypovolaemic – The body loses fluid, such as with major bleeds (internal and external), burns, diarrhoea and vomiting.

Cardiogenic – Heart attack - the heart is not pumping effectively.

Anaphylactic – The body reacts to something releasing large amounts of histamine and other hormones. These dilate the blood vessels and cause them to leak fluid, causing swelling of the airways and leading to a triple whammy of shock, affecting their airway, breathing and circulation.

Extremes of temperature can also cause the body to go into shock, as can a major assault on the nervous system such as a spinal or brain injury.

Symptoms of shock

Initially:

- Rapid pulse
- Pale, cold and clammy

As shock develops:

- Grey-blue skin colour and blue tinge to the lips - cyanosed
- Weak and dizzy
- Nausea and vomiting
- Thirst
- Shallow, rapid breathing

As the brain is struggling for oxygen:

- They may become restless and possibly aggressive - a sense of 'impending doom'.
- They may begin yawning and gasping for air.
- Eventually they will lose consciousness and become unresponsive and finally stop breathing.

Treatment of shock

If the shock is due to a major bleed, apply pressure to the wound and get them to lie down and raise their legs.

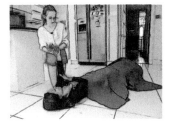

If you suspect the shock is caused by a heart attack, put them in the lazy W position. If they have a severe head injury or you are worried about their spine, keep them still, support their head and neck and avoid them twisting their spine.

Shock is made worse when someone is cold, anxious and in pain, reassuring them and keeping them warm can make a real difference.

Call an ambulance

Moisten their lips if they are complaining of thirst. **Do not give them a drink,** as they may need an operation and it is safer to give someone a general anaesthetic when they have an empty stomach.

Internal bleeding

Internal bleeding can be difficult to diagnose. The body can lose large amounts of blood from a ruptured organ, major fracture or stabbing which on the surface does not look too serious.

Key signs of internal bleeding

- Pale, cold, clammy, feeling sick and thirsty
- Possible bruising
- Chest pain or abdominal pain
- Swelling in the affected area
- Seepage from orifices - this may be discovered by the casualty or later in a medical environment. A first aider should not be looking for blood loss in any intimate areas.

Call an ambulance

If they show signs of shock, position them in the best position to increase the blood flow to the heart and brain - this is usually lying down with their legs raised, and cover them with a blanket.

Fainting

Fainting is a brief loss of consciousness caused by a temporary reduction to the blood flow of the brain.

Fainting can be a reaction to pain, lack of food, exhaustion or emotional stress. People often feel faint because it is warm or they have been exercising and then stop. The small blood vessels in their skin become dilated and the blood begins to pool in their feet. Lying down and raising the legs will improve the circulation and redirect the blood to the brain. They should feel better or come round quickly but if they don't, you will need to put them into the recovery position.

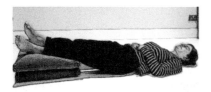

If it is really warm there is no need to cover them.

Lie them down and raise their legs.

Bites and Stings

Tick bites

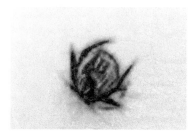

Ticks are tiny creatures that live in woodland and grassy areas. They are particularly prevalent if there are deer and other wildlife. They are blood sucking and bite into the skin to feed on blood. Initially, they are extremely small, but swell as they eat, eventually becoming pea-sized and therefore easier to spot and remove.

Ticks can carry Lyme disease and should ideally be removed by a medical professional. If this is not possible, they should be very carefully removed with tweezers or ideally with a proper tick remover, gently pulling without twisting in any way. When using a tick remover, you should insert under the tick and rotate 360 degrees. It is possible for the tick to be only half removed and to leave its mouthparts in the skin; this can lead to infection, which will need medical treatment and possibly antibiotics.

Never burn the tick off, or try and use chemicals to kill it. Keep the tick in a container to show to the medical professionals so they can ensure it has been removed entirely.

Cover up when walking in woodland and long grasses and always check yourself, your clothes and your dog on your return.

Lyme disease

Lyme disease is a serious illness in humans, characterised by flu like symptoms, lethargy and aches and pains. 50% of people with Lyme disease develop a classic bull's eye rash, which can appear on any part of the body and not necessarily where they were bitten. If you are worried you might have contracted Lyme disease, visit your doctor urgently. If Lyme disease is diagnosed and treated quickly, it is possible to make a full recovery. However, it can cause paralysis, arthritis, meningitis and severe long term problems.

Never burn the tick off, or try and use chemicals to kill it. Keep the tick in a container to show to the medical professionals so they can ensure it has been removed entirely.

Snake bite

The adder is the only poisonous snake in the wild in the UK. However, some venomous exotic snakes are kept as pets and we might also come across them when we are on holiday.

Recognizing that someone has been bitten

- There may be a pair of puncture marks
- Severe pain and redness around the puncture site
- Early signs of allergic reaction and anaphylaxis
- Nausea and vomiting
- Difficulty focusing
- Breathlessness, possible loss of consciousness and they could stop breathing

What to do

- Reassure the casualty and encourage them to keep still to slow the spread of the venom
- Phone for an ambulance
- Carefully wash the wound with water

Bandage the whole limb, immobilise and keep below the level of the heart

- Firmly bandage from just above the wound down the whole length of the limb, ensuring there is still circulation to the fingers or toes. Loosen if they experience numbness or tingling.

- Splint or immobilize the wound if possible to prevent moving the venom around the blood stream. This can be done with a stick or something to splint it, or if it is a leg that has been bitten, by bandaging the 2 legs together. Ensure there is adequate padding between them.

- Keep the wound below the level of the heart.

- If they show signs of anaphylaxis, treat appropriately.

- If they stop breathing - start CPR.

NEVER use a tourniquet as this will cut off the blood supply to the whole limb and is likely to make things worse.

Tip - If you have seen the snake, it is helpful to try and remember its markings and head shape to describe to the medical professionals.

Animal bites

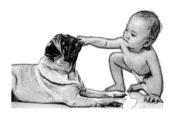

Never leave a child on their own with a pet, as children are often bitten on the face. Be sensitive to your pet's moods as even the tamest family pet can have a bad day!

Bites from animals can be jagged and frequently get infected. Even if an animal bite has just punctured the skin, it is important to wash the wound really well and look out for any signs of infection. It is sensible to get any bite that has punctured the skin looked at by a medical professional. If the wound looks red and becomes inflamed, hot, or angry looking, it is getting infected and the casualty will need antibiotics.

Treating the bite

The steps in treating the bite are as follows:

- Reassure the casualty
- Wash the wound thoroughly with clean water (and antibacterial soap depending on the location of the wound)
- Stop any bleeding
- Elevate the wound and apply pressure to stop bleeding
- Be ready to treat for shockBe ready to treat for shock

- **Note:** Outside the UK, if someone is bitten or licked in a wound, it is important to get medical attention very fast and have anti-rabies medication. It is also important to ensure that they are covered for tetanus.

Bee stings

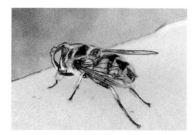

Bee stings - if someone is stung by a bee and the sting is still in the skin, quickly flick it out using your thumb nail or a credit card. It is important not to squeeze the sting as this can increase the amount of allergen entering the body and can increase any possible allergic reaction. Wasps and other stinging insects do not leave the sting behind in the wound.

If the casualty has a local reaction, a wrapped ice pack applied to the area can quickly help to reduce the swelling. Piriton (an antihistamine) is also helpful (children should only be given medication with prior written approval from their parents).

Oral antihistamine takes about 15 minutes to work

If the casualty shows any signs of a systemic reaction or of anaphylactic shock, call an ambulance immediately and use their adrenaline auto-injector if they have been prescribed one. Reassuring them and positioning them appropriately can make a major difference to their treatment.

If someone is very short of breath, they should be encouraged to sit in an upright position to help their breathing. Putting something under their knees to help increase their circulation can be very helpful.

If they are not having difficulty breathing, but are pale, cold, clammy, feeling sick and thirsty - they should lie down with their legs raised to help increase the circulation to their vital organs. Encourage them to turn their head to one side if they are likely to vomit. They should be covered to keep them warm and remain in this position until the paramedics arrive.

Marine stings

Basic safety when playing at the beach, paddling and snorkelling is important. Children should wear beach shoes when paddling and swimming as Weever fish and sea urchin spines can easily get embedded if they are accidentally trodden on.

Jelly fish stings

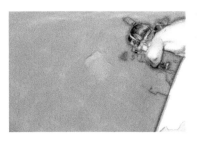

- Reassure the casualty and sit them down
- If there are any tentacles remaining, remove with tweezers - get a medical professional to do this if you are unsure
- If they show any signs of breathing problems, or acute allergic reaction or anaphylaxis, phone an ambulance immediately
- Soak the affected area in vinegar for 15-30 minutes

NOTE - with stings from a Portuguese Man of War (these are not jellyfish but are often mistaken for them) - do not immerse in vinegar as it will make the pain worse.

Sea urchins and Weever fish

Sea urchins and Weever fish both have vicious spines that can easily get embedded and can break off leaving the tip deep in the skin.

- Soak the area in as hot water as possible ensuring that you are not scalding the casualty.
- Remove large spines with tweezers, being careful not to snap them.
- Look out for any signs of local or systemic reaction - if there are signs of anaphylaxis treat appropriately.

Do not cover the wound and keep checking on it - if there is severe redness or swelling it may be starting to get infected and they might need antibiotics.

Burns

Prevention is key

Babies and small children have extremely sensitive skin. They can be burnt with a hot drink that is at drinking temperature for an adult. As people get older, their skin becomes thinner and more prone to burns.

Be extremely careful with hot drinks. Never pass them over the top of other people; always keep hot drinks out of the reach of babies and children, and never drink a hot drink when you are holding a child.

For toddlers and small children, be particularly vigilant about keeping them safe from dishwasher tablets, other chemicals, button batteries, electrical wires and over hanging flexes.

Fit a thermostat to the bath tap to ensure that the water remains at a constant temperature and protect from frightening fluctuations.

Overview as to how to treat a burn

For all burns - treat immediately with cool, running water.

- Carefully remove any loose clothing covering the burn.

Do **not** remove clothes if there is any risk the skin has stuck to them or if the skin has blistered.

- Put the affected area under cool running water for at least 10 minutes. Remember you are cooling the burn and not the casualty.
- Keep the casualty warm and dry and look for early signs of shock.
- Phone an ambulance, particularly if a large area is affected, or if the skin is broken or blistered and keep the area under cool running water while you are waiting for the paramedics to arrive.

For a burn from a flame - stop, drop, cover and roll to extinguish the fire and then treat under cool running water.

Causes of burns

A burn can be caused by many different things:

- Steam
- Flames
- Hot liquids
- Friction
- Hot objects such as irons, electric hobs, heated towel rails
- Ice and extremely cold objects
- Chemicals
- Sun lamps

If the burn is caused by a **chemical**, run under cool running water for at least 20 minutes and be careful of the run-off as it could still be corrosive and hurt you. Look at the advice on the packaging and see if there are any specific instructions.

Sunburn

Prevent sunburn by avoiding the midday heat and wearing sun cream, hats and sun-resistant material.

If a baby or small child has been sunburnt, it is likely that they will also be suffering from heat exhaustion and you should always seek medical help. Cool the affected area and give them plenty to drink to rehydrate them.

For an older child or adult:

- Cool the area under a shower for at least 10 minutes, or apply repeated cool wet towels for 15 minutes.

- When completely cooled, apply neat aloe vera gel to the affected area. This will soothe, reduce swelling and promote healing.

- Give the casualty plenty to drink and seek medical advice. If a baby or small child has experienced sunburn, always look for signs of heat exhaustion and get medical advice.

Electrical burns

It is extremely difficult to electrocute yourself in a UK socket. However, babies have little fingers and have time. It is more common for a wire to have become damaged and frayed and when it is touched, the baby or child receives an electric shock. It is possible that if they grasp the damaged flex, the current will prevent them from letting go of the wire.

If you go to help someone who is holding onto an electrical wire with the current through them, you can be electrocuted too. It is therefore vital that you know where the electricity mains is situated and how to turn it off.

If someone has been electrocuted

Do not touch them until you have turned the electricity off at the mains. Electrical burns have an entry and exit and burn all the way through the inside. Therefore, the electrical burn is unlikely to be the most important injury and should not be a distraction when someone may be losing consciousness and could stop breathing because of the shock affecting their heart.

Size, Cause, Age, Location, Depth

Size – the larger the area involved, the more serious it is for the casualty and the more likely they are to suffer from shock.

Cause – a burn can be caused by many different things.

Age – burns are more serious in babies and children and the elderly.

Location – burns to the hands, face, feet, genitals, airways, or a burn that extends all the way around a limb, are particularly serious. Keep the burnt area under cool running water until the paramedic arrives.

Depth –superficial, partial thickness or full thickness burns.

All burns are serious, and particularly so when it is a child or someone elderly who is burnt. Often people have different depths of burn within a single injury. Whatever the depth of burn, they should all be treated under cool running water.

Determining the depth of the burn

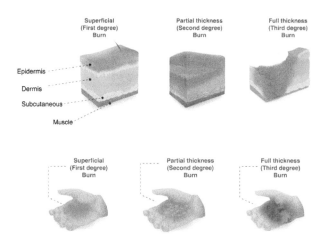

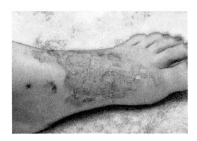

A superficial burn has just affected the top layer of skin. It is really painful and likely to blister.

Thickness of the burn

A partial thickness burn is really painful. The burn has gone through both the first and second layer of skin.

Full thickness burns are often not as painful as the nerves have been severely damaged too. This is the most severe sort of burn, the skin may appear pale, white or charred it will require extensive treatment and skin grafts.

Treating a burn

Treating a burn promptly under cool running water for at least 10 minutes makes a huge difference to the severity of a burn and therefore the amount of pain, scarring, length of time in hospital that the casualty may experience.

Never touch the burn, pop blisters, or put on any creams whatsoever. Take burns very seriously and always seek medical advice.

Wear sterile gloves when dealing with burns.

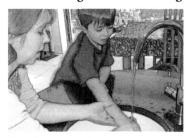

Cool the burn under cool running water (keeping the casualty warm).

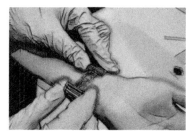

Remove any watches, jewellery, etc and loosen clothing.

If a baby, child or elderly person is burnt, phone for an ambulance and keep cooling their burn under cool running water.

Scalds

Scalds are burns caused by hot liquids. The hot liquid can continue to burn through the clothes, so it is important to remove any loose clothing and cool the burn thoroughly as quickly as possible.

Always be particularly vigilant about hot drinks as baby's skin is more sensitive than an adult's and they can be burnt by a drink that has been standing for many minutes.

There was a baby in the burns unit who had been in a coffee shop when a cup of hot coffee was passed over them and it spilt on their arm. They were swiftly treated under cool running water and their arm was ok. Unfortunately, no-one had noticed that the coffee had also been spilt on their foot. They were wearing fur lined baby boots. Everyone was so busy attending to the obvious arm injury, that by the time they noticed the foot, it was badly blistered and needed hospitalisation.

Always check anywhere else that the hot liquid might have splashed or spilt.

Treatment for scalds

- **Remove clothing** - if sure it has not stuck.

- **Cool** - for at least 10 minutes.

- **Get medical advice** - once cooled it can be dressed with a proper burnsdressing, cling film or clean plastic bag.

- Do not touch the burn - wear sterile gloves if possible.

Dressing a burn

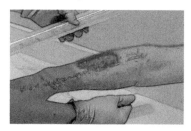

A burn should not be dressed until it has been cooled for at least 15 minutes. Covering a burn reduces the risk of infection and reduces pain by covering exposed nerve endings.

If a person is burnt and the burn is bad enough that you need to dress it, phone an ambulance while continuing to cool it under running water. The paramedics will dress it for you.

If you want to dress the burn, cling film is a good temporary dressing. Ensure you have cooled the burn for at least 15 minutes before dressing it. Discard the first couple of turns of cling film and place an inner piece loosely over the burn. Plastic bags and non-fluffy dressings also make useful dressings. Proper burns dressings are great, but ideally the burn should be cooled for at least 10 minutes before dressing.

Always get a medical professional to assess a burn

Never:

- Remove anything that has stuck to a burn

- Touch a burn

- Burst blisters

- Apply any creams, lotions or fats

- Apply tight dressings, tapes or use anything fluffy

Inhalation of fumes

- Take the person away from the smoke and encourage them to breathe fresh air if possible.

- Check consciousness, airway and breathing and be prepared to resuscitate if necessary.

- Burns to the airway need to be treated as an urgent medical emergency and you will need an ambulance. They may have difficulty breathing, be slightly blue around the lips, have soot around their mouth and could have a hoarse voice and painful throat. If they are fully conscious, sitting them upright to help their breathing and giving them small sips of cool water is helpful. Do not leave them, and continually reassess them to check they are not losing consciousness.

Please note that carbon monoxide is a silent killer. There is no smell associated with it and it is vitally important to have appliances checked regularly and to fit a carbon monoxide detector.

Poisoning

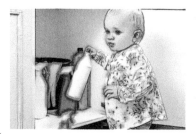

A poison is any substance (a solid, liquid, or a gas) which can cause damage if it enters the body in sufficient quantities.

A poison can be swallowed, breathed in, absorbed through the skin or injected.

Some poisons cause an all-over reaction and can result in seizures, blurred vision, acute anaphylaxis and can be fatal. Be cautious and always get the casualty quickly seen by a medical professional.

If you suspect that someone has taken a harmful substance, call an ambulance and explain clearly what has happened. They will advise you what to do.

The following advice is relevant to anyone who has been exposed to, or taken a poisonous substance, either accidentally or on purpose:

- Keep all potentially harmful substances out of reach of small children and ideally in a locked cupboard. This includes; dishwasher tablets, medicines, alcohol, cosmetics, DIY, cleaning and gardening products and potentially poisonous plants.

- Ensure that grandparents, child carers and visitors are also mindful about leaving potentially hazardous substances within reach; the contents of many handbags could be fascinating and lethal to a small child.

- Never decant medication or any other products into different containers.

- Always use the original containers, clearly labelled, ideally with childproof lids.

- Ensure people needing to take numerous pills are competent with their medication. Pharmacists can help by supplying pre-prepared pill boxes to make it easier for people to take the right medication at the prescribed times.

- Keep batteries out of reach of small children and ensure that batteries in their toys are firmly secured.

- Fit carbon monoxide alarms and have appliances and alarms regularly checked.

- Tidy up straight after a party if there are children in the house. Otherwise little ones are likely to be the first up and may well finish the dregs of the drinks and help themselves to anything else available before you emerge.

- Be aware of harmful plants - many decorative plants (particularly berry bearing Christmas plants) are toxic. Plants can be checked through the Royal Horticultural Society (rhs.org.uk) or by asking your local florist or horticultural nursery.

Poisoning from an ingested (swallowed) substance

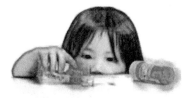

This topic relates to anyone of any age who you suspect may have accidentally or purposefully taken a potentially harmful substance.

Should you find a child occupied with something potentially dangerous and be unsure if they have taken anything, always get them checked.

Depending on what they have taken, they could have a burning sensation of their lips and mouth, nausea or vomiting, drowsiness or hyper-mania and possibly a change in their heartbeat.

If someone has swallowed a non-corrosive substance (a product that will not burn them) and if they appear completely well:

- Encourage them to stay still, as moving around will increase their metabolism and speed up the poison circulating around their body.

- Calmly encourage them to tell you what has happened (they may not tell you if they are scared or feel you are angry).

- If they appear fine, phone 111 or the Poisons Unit and get advice from them.

- If the casualty becomes unconscious, open the airway and check for breathing. Be ready to resuscitate if necessary - and use a protective face shield to ensure you don't put yourself at risk from whatever they have taken.

Tip: If a child has swallowed a berry from a plant - take a photo of the plant and a leaf as well, both of these will help the medical team to identify the berry and establish whether it is harmful or not.

If someone has swallowed a corrosive or burning substance

If a child was to mistake a dishwasher or washing machine capsule or tablet for a sweet, it could prove fatal - cleaning products are extremely alkaline and can burn the skin or throat.

IIf someone has bitten a dishwasher capsule:

- Stay as calm as you can.

- Remove it and rinse the product away as quickly as you can. Protect yourself if possible, but attend to them fast.

If they have swallowed some of the product:

- Ideally get them to swill milk or water around their mouth and spit it out to remove as much as possible and then give small sips of milk or water to dilute the product further down their throat.

Do not make them sick as this will cause them to burn again as the corrosive product comes back up.

Phone for an ambulance and keep giving them small sips of milk or water.

Look at the box that the substance has come from and read the advice in case of accidental ingestion.

If they have swallowed the product, it is possible that it will have burnt both their oesophagus and their airway and this can lead to their airway swelling and becoming obstructed so that they are unable to breathe. If this happens and they become unconscious and stop breathing, you will need to resuscitate them by giving them CPR.

It is important that you protect yourself when giving the breaths - this can be done with a pocket mask or face shield, if you have one available - thereby protecting yourself and ensuring that you are not burnt as well. If you don't have a face shield or anything suitable to use, do not put yourself at risk and if necessary, just give compressions.

When you go to hospital, take the packaging and the remains of anything you think they may have swallowed as this will help the doctors to treat them in the best way possible.

Breaks, sprains and dislocations

How do you know if they have broken a bone?

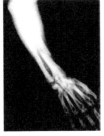

The honest answer is that unless the bone is sticking out, or the limb is at a very peculiar angle, the only way to know for sure that a bone is broken is to have an x-ray.

A fracture is another word for a broken bone.

Broken bones on their own rarely cause fatalities. However, particularly if there is bleeding associated with the injury (either internal or external bleeding) this can cause the casualty to go into shock, which is life threatening. Keep the casualty warm and dry and be aware that pain and stress will adversely affect their condition. If you are at all worried about them, phone an ambulance.

Types of fractures

Open fractures

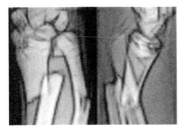

If the bone is sticking out, the bone is broken!

Your priority is to stop bleeding without pushing on the bone or moving the broken bone at all and then get emergency help.

Be very aware of the onset of shock. Keep them warm and dry; if they show any signs of shock, lie them down, but do not elevate the injured limb.

Complicated fractures

With complicated fractures, muscles, nerves, tendons and blood vessels could be trapped and damaged. If you are aware that they have lost feeling in part of their limb, or if it has changed colour, they will need urgent medical treatment.

Keep them calm, warm and supported, and phone for an ambulance.

Closed fractures

With a closed fracture, the bone has not come through the skin. Children commonly have greenstick fractures, where the bone doesn't snap, but half breaks like a spring stick.

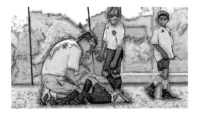

For all possible closed fractures and soft tissue injuries you should initially do the following:

- **P**rotect the injury (stop using the injured limb, pad to protect)
- **R**est the injury
- **I**ce - apply a wrapped ice pack
- **C**omfortable support - apply a supportive bandage
- **E**levate - to reduce swelling.

You will need to get them to hospital for an x-ray to establish whether it is broken or whether it is a soft tissue injury.

Call an ambulance if:

- They start to show signs of shock
- There is a possibility that they have injured their spine or head
- They have any difficulty breathing or begin to lose consciousness
- It is an open fracture, with the bone through the skin
- If they lose feeling in the limb, or if it dramatically changes colour
- You are unable to safely transport the child to hospital yourself
- There is a suspected pelvic or hip fracture
- You are worried about them in any way

Dislocation

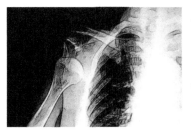

A dislocation occurs when the bone is pulled out of position at a joint and is often accompanied by other tissue damage.

Always get a medical professional to put a dislocated joint back as you could cause further damage and trap nerves or blood vessels trying to put it back yourself.

Signs and symptoms of a dislocated joint

- Difficulty moving the joint, pain and stiffness

- Swelling and bruising around the joint

- Asymmetry, with one joint looking deformed and out of place

- Shortening, bending or twisting of the joint

Treatment

- Support the injury to avoid unnecessary and painful movement (the casualty may prefer to do this themselves).

Never try and reposition the limb yourself. Look out for signs of shock and transport them to hospital or phone an ambulance. Do not allow them to eat or drink as they may need a general anaesthetic.

If someone has dislocated their jaw, do not bandage the jaw as this could be very dangerous; get them to support their lower jaw by cupping it in their hands and get them to hospital.

Bandaging

If you are bandaging a joint, you should always go from half way down eachlimb, rather than just bandaging the joint as this can cut off the circulation. Bandage firmly, but not too tightly, overlapping half the bandage each turn.

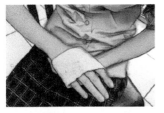

Press on the nail bed to ensure that the colour comes back immediately, demonstrating that you have not applied the bandage too tightly.

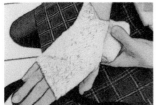

To bandage someone's wrist, start at the base of the fingers (do the same for an ankle, starting near the toes).

Wrap the bandage round, overlapping by half a bandage width each time.

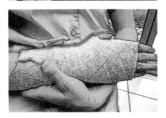

Support the arm in a broad arm sling, if the casualty would like you to do this. They may prefer to hold it themselves.

Slings

A broad arm sling to support a sprained wrist

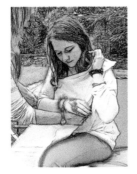

If the child prefers to hold the injured limb himself and not to have a sling, that is fine. You can also offer additional support by creating an improvised sling using clothes - such as pinning their coat sleeve to their shoulder, turning up the hem of their jumper or partbuttoning their coat to enable them to support their hand between the buttons.

Encourage the casualty to support their own wrist.

Use a triangular bandage; put it under the injured arm with the 90 degree corner to the elbow. Slip under the injured arm to support it and wrap over the top, securing the sling on the neck. (For a small child, the triangular bandage can be folded in half first). Tie a knot to support the sling.

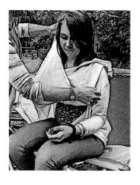 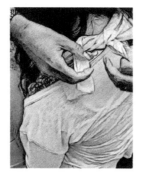 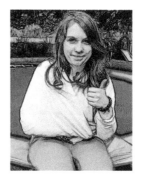

Tie a reef knot or secure flat knot to support the sling in position.

Secure the corner at the elbow by twisting and tucking it in, or fastening with a safety pin or tape.

Head injuries

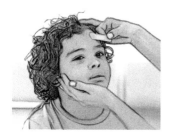

Anyone who has a knock to the head needs to be aware of the signs and symptoms of concussion and compression.

Someone who has sustained a head injury should ideally not be left on their own for the next 48 hours and should refrain from driving until they have been fully assessed.

It can be difficult to tell whether a head injury is serious or not. Most head injuries simply result in a superficial bump or bruise, but severe, or repeated head injuries can result in damage to the brain.

Fortunately, most falls or blows to the head result in injury to the scalp only, which is usually more frightening than life threatening - the head and face are very vascular and consequently injuries bleed profusely and can be very scary!

An internal head injury may have more serious implications because it could cause damage to the brain. An internal head injury may become apparent immediately or up to a couple of days after the accident. The casualty should be observed closely over the next few days and if you see anything unusual, you should seek medical attention immediately.

Remember: a serious head injury can also result in a spinal injury due to the whiplash effect.

If in any doubt, get medical attention. In hospital, if they are concerned, they will do a CT scan to establish the extent of the injury.

What to look for and what to do

If a baby has more than a very minor head injury, call an ambulance immediately. Also call an ambulance if a child has lost consciousness, even momentarily, or if a casualty of any age has any of these symptoms:

- Complains of head and neck pain
- Isn't walking normally

For everyone else (other than babies and anyone who has lost consciousness), if they are alert and behaving normally after the fall or blow:

- Talk to the casualty and check that they are fully alert and orientated (know where they are and what happened).
- Apply a wrapped ice pack or instant cold pack to the injured area for 10 minutes.
- Observe them carefully for the next 24 hours. If you notice anything unusual, phone an ambulance immediately.

If the incident has occurred with a child close to bedtime or naptime and they fall asleep soon afterwards, check in every few hours and look out for twitching limbs or disturbances in colour or strange breathing.

It is perfectly ok for your child to go to sleep providing you are certain that they are behaving normally and there are no unusual signs or symptoms. There is no need to keep a child awake after a head injury.

If you aren't comfortable with your child's appearance (trust your instincts), rouse your child. They should object to this and attempt to resettle. If he or she doesn't protest, try to wake them fully. If your child can't be woken, or shows any symptoms of a brain injury (see below) call an ambulance immediately.

Compression and concussion

If the brain is injured, it will swell and may bleed, as with an injury to any other part of the body. However, as the brain is contained within the skull; it can only press against other parts of the brain and against the spinal cord. This results in compression of these vital organs and can be fatal. Compression can happen almost immediately, or up to 48 hours after the bang on the head and even longer if they hit their head again.

Look out for anything unusual.

Concussion

Concussion is a reversible form of brain injury. Following a severe blow to the head, it is usual to experience pain, possible short term loss of memory, dizziness and confusion. Someone with concussion should always be monitored to check for signs of compression. If you see anything unusual at all or are worried about their condition, you should phone for an ambulance.

Do not leave anyone who has had a severe head injury on their own - they should have a responsible adult with them who understands the signs of brain injury and what to look out for. When looking after children, you should ensure that all carers are aware that the child has hit their head. The child should ideally sleep in the same room as their parents for the next couple of nights.

When to call an ambulance following a serious head injury

Call an ambulance if someone has a head injury and any one of the following symptoms:

- Unconsciousness

- Abnormal breathing

- Obvious serious wound or suspected skull fracture

- Bleeding or clear fluid from the nose, ear, or mouth
- Lack of co-ordination
- Disturbance of speech or vision
- Pupils of unequal size
- Weakness or paralysis
- Dizziness
- Neck pain or stiffness
- Fitting
- Vomiting

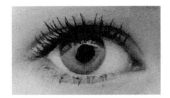 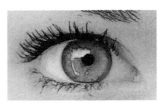

Dilated Pupil   Constricted Pupils

If someone is unconscious:

- If they are breathing - roll them into the recovery position (on their side so that their tongue falls forward in their mouth and any vomit can drain away), trying not to twist their neck or spine at all. Any head injury may well have caused spinal damage as the head recoils from the blow.
- If they are not breathing, start CPR.
- Call for an ambulance.

If someone is conscious and it is a serious head injury:

- Phone for an ambulance.
- Do your best to keep the casualty calm and still - making sure that they do not twist as they could have a spinal injury.
- If there is bleeding, grab a clean cloth and apply pressure.
- Do not attempt to clean the wound as it could make things worse.
- Do not apply forceful direct pressure to the wound if you suspect the skull is fractured.

- Do not remove any object that's stuck in the wound.

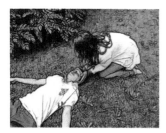

Support their head and neck, without covering their ears so they can hear you, keeping their spine in line and encourage them not to twist.

Remember: a serious head injury can also result in a spinal injury due to the whiplash effect.

Concussion - get medical advice	Compression -999/112 immediately
Could be unconciousness for a short period and then recovers quickly	Head injury: may appear to recover but then deteriorates. **Can happen immediately or up to 48 hours after**
Short term memory loss (particularly of the incident). **Could be confused and irritable.**	Levels of response become worse as condition develops
Headache	Intense headache
Pale, clammy skin	Flushed, dry skin
Shallow, normal breathing	Deep, noisy, slow breathing. *Pressure on the respiratory center of the brain*
Rapid, weak pulse. *Blood diverts away from the extremities*	Slow, strong pulse. *Caused by raised blood pressure*
Normal pupils, reacting to light	One or both pupils dilate as pressure increases on the brain
Possible nausea or vomiting on recovery	Condition becomes worse. Could start fitting. **Call an ambulance**

What to look out for following a head injury

The brain is cushioned by cerebrospinal fluid, but a severe blow to the head may knock the brain into the side of the skull or tear blood vessels – like a jelly in a box. Any internal head injury — fractured skull, torn blood vessels, or damage to the brain itself — can cause the brain to swell. This can be serious and possibly life threatening.

Signs and symptoms to look out for following a head injury

The following signs and symptoms can appear immediately or over the next couple of days. Keep a close eye on the casualty and get medical advice if at all concerned.

Observed by others

- Appears stunned or dazed

- Loses consciousness (even briefly)

- Is confused about events

- Trouble thinking or concentrating

- Can't recall events prior or after event

- Shows behaviour or personality changes

- Answer questions slowly and repeats questions

- Has difficulty remembering things and organising themselves

Experienced by casualty

- Headache or pressure in the head

- Balance problems or dizziness

- Nausea/vomiting

- Sensitivity to light or noise

- Does not feel right

- Blurred vision or double vision

- Feel "dazed", sluggish, foggy or groggy

- Difficulty concentrating or remembering

- Feeling irritable, sad, nervous or more emotional

- Sleep disturbances

Different levels of injury require different levels of concern. It can be difficult to determine the level of injury, so it's always wise to discuss a head injury with your doctor. A clear indicator of a more serious injury is when someone loses consciousness or is confused.

These symptoms can come on at any time from immediately after the accident to a couple of days later.

Skull fracture

You should suspect a skull fracture if:

- They have watery blood coming from their ears or nose

- They have bruising around their eyes, or behind an ear

- There's an open wound on their head

If they are conscious:

- Keep them as still as you can and don't let them twist as they could well have a spinal injury.

- Get the emergency services on their way immediately.

If they are unresponsive and breathing normally:

- Put them into the recovery position.

- Protect their spine and do your best not to let them twist.

- If they are unconscious and not breathing, start CPR.

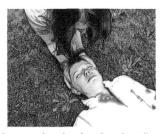

Support their head and neck without covering their ears

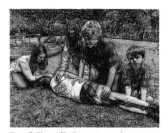

Carefully roll them into the recovery position keeping their spine straight.

Keep supporting their head and neck - do not let go until the paramedics are able to take over.

Special consideration

If you have a casualty who is unresponsive and breathing and you are worried about the possibility that they have a spinal injury; if you have been trained to recognise early signs of airway obstruction and are confident in doing so; keep the casualty in the position that they have landed in and support their head and neck using MILS (manual in-line stabilisation) and get someone to phone an ambulance immediately.

If you are at all concerned about their airway, put them into the recovery position immediately, monitoring their breathing continually.

Head injury advice - when to play on

We have all witnessed the inevitable clash of heads during a match and the dilemma of the coach and match officials to do the right thing. This uncertainty is compounded by the player, pumped full of match adrenaline, desperately trying to hide the extent of the head injury to be able to play on. The RFU guidance makes it easier for everyone to do the right thing and ensure the player has every opportunity to make a full recovery.

Concussion is a disturbance to the normal working of the brain usually resulting from a blow to the head. Repeated concussions are linked to serious long term brain conditions.

Initial symptoms of concussion - in rugby the most common symptoms that you may see on the pitch are the following: headache, confusion, blurred vision, nausea, difficulty concentrating, fatigue, drowsiness, dizziness, feeling in a fog, memory impairment. Concussion can also affect someone's mood, balance, sleep, thinking, concentration and senses. Most symptoms resolve in 7-10 days and many much sooner.

It is important to realise that concussion is an injury to the brain and this injury needs to be rested to fully recover, in a similar way to that of a sprain or strain. The injury to the brain occurs during the collision, when the brain is shaken within the skull. If someone rests appropriately following concussion, they will nearly always make a full recovery.

Most important advice following a head injury

- Don't make things worse - it's important to take it seriously and rest.

- Do not risk recurring injury.

- Rest your brain: lots of sleep, avoid reading, screens and sports for at least 24 hours/48 hours for child.

Children and adolescents may need one or 2 days off school and a gradual return to academic study. They can start light reading and small amounts of screen time, but should stop if there are signs of any recurrence of symptoms.

Those who play sports should take at least 2 weeks with no training to give the brain a chance to fully recover.

If there are no symptoms, players can then start the gradual return to play:

24 hours per stage (48 hours for children and adolescents) - go back a stage if symptoms occur.

1. Light aerobic exercise

2. Sport specific exercise

3. Non-contact training

4. Full contact practice

19 days is the earliest that an adult can return to play.

23 days is the earliest that a child or adolescent can return to play.

Repeated concussions, particularly in children, are associated with long term consequences and serious conditions including second impact syndrome and postconcussion syndrome.

Coaches and first aiders should be confident to:

Remove - any player who has experienced a head injury and shows any of the above symptoms should be removed from play immediately.

Recognise - learn the signs of concussion. Only about 10% of people experiencing concussion are knocked out - so 90% of people who have experienced concussion will remain conscious. Look out for the more obvious signs such as a dazed or blank expression or tonic arm extension following the blow to the head, along with the symptoms listed above. Use the pocket concussion assessment tool available from the RFU.

Applying a wrapped ice pack will reduce superficial bruising and swelling, but this has no effect on any brain recovery.

If a severe head injury has been sustained and you are concerned about the casualty's spine, they should only be removed from the field by someone appropriately trained to do so. If you're worried and there's no one appropriate to help, reassure the casualty, support their head in a neutral position, stop the game - or move to another pitch and await removal of the casualty by paramedics.

- **Rest** - for at least 24 hours for an adult and 48 for a child or adolescent (see above).
- **Recover** - ensure the player remains completely symptom free before contemplating any form of return to play.
- **Return** - return to play using the gradual return to play (GRTP) method as outlined above.

IIt may take 4-6 weeks before a player is fully fit and back to competitive play. This may seem a long time away from the game. However, it is comparable to the recovery time following a soft tissue injury and your brain is so important to every aspect of life that it is vital we take head injuries seriously.

The RFU have superb online training courses specific to parents, players, teachers and coaches.
http://www.englandrugby.com/my-rugby/players/player-health concussion-headcase/

Spinal injuries

You should consider the possibility of a spinal injury if:

- The casualty has fallen from more than twice their height, or been pushed with force.

- Something heavy has fallen onto them.

- They have been involved in a road traffic accident – either within a moving vehicle, or being hit by anything at speed, particularly if it is over 15 mph.

- They have been doing any form of combat or contact sport.

- They have a head injury.

- If they are conscious, encourage them to remain completely still, but do not restrain them. You want to avoid them twisting.

How to log roll someone into the recovery position

If they are unresponsive but breathing, you will need to carefully put them into the recovery position, ideally by log rolling.

Most people don't have spinal injuries, but it is important to be cautious. It is possible to have broken your back or neck and not know; it is not until it is x-rayed that the break is discovered. It is vital to keep the spine in-line and avoid them twisting.

If they have a damaged spinal column (bones) and twist, it can damage the spinal cord and result in paralysis.

Shout to them to keep still and tell them you are coming over.

Support their head and neck in-line with the body, whilst you assess their level of consciousness. DO NOT MOVE THEM! Get someone to phone for an ambulance.

Support their head and neck, but don't cover their ears, as hearing is the last sense to go and the first to come back.

To assess their level of consciousness, first speak to them. Clearly tell them who you are and ask if they are okay or if they can open their eyes. If there is no response, gently shake them, tap their shoulders or pinch their ears or nail bed.

If you get a response, you know they are alive and breathing.

If there is no response and they are breathing, they need to be put into the recovery position quickly and carefully.

To check if they are breathing, put your cheek above their mouth and nose, look down their body and look down the body, listen to their breathing and feel their breath on your cheek.

Keep supporting their head and neck. Very carefully straighten their limbs and quickly prepare to log roll them into the recovery position. Check the pocket on the side that you are rolling them onto.

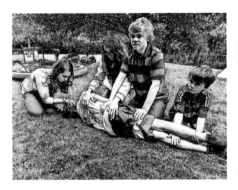

The second person, should position themselves at the shoulders and be ready to roll the casualty towards them.

The third person should position themselves in the middle of the body and overlap hands to support the casualty's body really well.

The fourth person supports the leg. They need to gutter the leg supporting underneath, so that when the casualty is rolled over, they remain as straight as possible without twisting their spine.

Check everyone is ready. The person holding the head should take charge. On the count of 3, everyone rolls together keeping the spine in line.

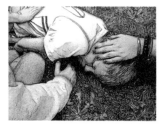

Check the casualty is over enough to keep the airway open and to allow the contents of their stomach to drain. **Keep supporting the head, do not let go until the paramedic takes over.** The other people should continue to support the lower part of the body. **Keep checking that they are breathing.**

Special consideration

If you have been trained to recognise the early recognition of airway obstruction and are confident in doing so, keep the casualty in the position they have landed in and support their head and neck using MILS (manual in-line stabilisation).

Also get someone to phone an ambulance immediately.

If you are at all concerned about their airway put them into the recovery position immediately, monitoring their breathing continually.

Support a casualty's head and neck if you suspect they could have a spinal injury.

Major crush injury – 15 minute rule

If someone is crushed by a heavy object

If you can safely remove the object within 15 minutes, you should do so. If a limb has been crushed for longer than 15 minutes – or if you are unsure how long they have been trapped - you should leave them as they are and get the emergency services on their way immediately.

If a limb has been deprived of blood supply for **longer than 15 minutes,** toxins start to build up and if the blood supply is suddenly restored by removing the heavy object, these toxins can swiftly circulate and cause a cardiac arrest.

Extreme caution should be taken with all serious crush injuries – if in doubt seek medical advice first.

Road traffic accidents

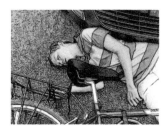

In most EU Countries, people learn first aid as part of their driving test, but this does not happen in the UK. Accidents happen and if involved in an accident it is a legal requirement to stop at the scene (only certain health professionals have a duty of care to help anyone who is injured). How many of us would know how to help someone injured on the road?

The following is a step-by-step guide, should you be the first on scene at an accident:

- When approaching an accident scene; the most important element is your safety. Make sure that all traffic has stopped and it is flagged up that there has been an accident. Otherwise there may be additional casualties.

- Be aware of oncoming traffic to ensure that it is not posing an additional danger. If there is any fuel spillage or potential fire risk, turn off car ignitions if possible. Put on hazard lights and encourage other cars to do the same. If you have anything fluorescent, wear it. Be bright and visible. Never put yourself at risk.

- If there are other people around, get them to phone the emergency services.

- Quickly establish how many vehicles have been involved and assess the occupants of all the vehicles to ensure no one has life-threatening injuries. People screaming, crying and making a noise are breathing – your initial priority is anyone quiet and not moving.

If anyone is not moving, quickly establish if they are responsive. If there is no response, check if they are breathing. If they are unresponsive and breathing, ensure they are in a position where they are leaning forward or to one side and are positioned so that the airway will remain open.

Move them as little as possible and avoid twisting them. Keep talking to the casualty calmly and explain what you are doing and why. The calmer everyone else will be. Also keep them warm and dry.

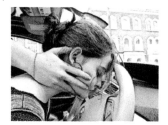

Support their head and neck and keep checking they are breathing. If the person is not breathing, you will need to resuscitate them – if you are on your own and have not called an ambulance make sure you do this now and ask their advice as to the best way to resuscitate, as this is not easy to do in a car.

Only remove an unconscious person from a vehicle if there is an immediate danger to their life from fire, flood, or an explosion. Ask the emergency services over the phone for their advice as to what you should do.

It is very difficult to extricate an unconscious person from a vehicle and there is a major danger that you could exacerbate their injuries and injure yourself in the process.

Conscious casualties should be entrusted to the care of bystanders and removed from the wreckage to a safe area. Be aware of confused and dazed casualties who may wander into danger. Brief the bystanders to keep the casualties warm and calm and help them to contact next of kin. Look for any major bleeding and life-threatening injuries and treat these.

Note the nature of the wreckage and be aware of possible injuries as a result: bodies are softer than metalwork, so if there is major damage to the vehicle it is possible that there could be internal injuries to the casualty. Ensure the bystanders notify you if there is any change in the casualty's condition.

Anyone trapped in a vehicle should be monitored carefully and the emergency services notified immediately. If someone is crushed, note the exact time when the accident happened as this is important in deciding on how and when to release the casualty.

If there are additional people around, show them how to support the person's neck to avoid them twisting, as there is the possibility of a spinal injury. If there is severe bleeding this will need to be controlled – wear gloves and apply dressings.

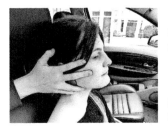

Support the head and neck to avoid them twisting, do not cover their ears, and keep talking to them calmly.

Do not allow anyone to smoke at the scene or give the casualties anything to eat or drink following the accident in case they later need an operation.

If a motorcyclist is involved, only remove their helmet if they are unconscious and there is no other way to assess their breathing or their airway is in danger. There is usually a way of lifting the visor, and it is sensible to loosen their chin strap.

If a casualty has been hit by a car and they are lying on their back unconscious and breathing, they should be carefully rolled into the recovery position to keep their spine in line.

This should ideally be done with the support of others to avoid twisting the spine. (If you have received advanced training on MILS (Manual In-Line Stabilisation) and are confident that you can react quickly if their airway is in danger – then maintain MILS and continuous airway monitoring and roll them into the recovery position immediately should they begin to obstruct).

If a casualty has been hit by a vehicle or thrown from one and they are conscious in the road, they should be encouraged to keep still. Ensure that someone is directing traffic and maintaining safety.

Support their head and neck, keep them warm and dry and wait for the emergency services.

Fitting/Seizures/Convulsions

What is a seizure?

1 in 20 people will experience some sort of a seizure during their lives.

A seizure (the medical term for a fit or convulsion) occurs when there is a sudden burst of electrical activity in the brain which temporarily interferes with the normal messaging processes.

Seizures can be focal (partial) when only one part of the brain is affected, or generalised when both sides of the brain are involved. Sometimes a seizure can start as focal and then develop into a more complex generalised one.

Focal (partial) seizures

These can affect a large part of one hemisphere or just a small area in one of the lobes. What happens during the seizure will depend on where in the brain the seizure happens and what that part of the brain usually does. Therefore, it can be helpful to observe someone while they are having a seizure as it can help neurologists identify what part of the brain is affected. Often the person having a seizure remains conscious but experiences a strange sensation, rigidity of their muscles and confusion.

General seizures

Generalised seizures affect both sides of the brain at once and can happen without warning, sometimes occurring straight after a focal seizure. The person is likely to lose consciousness, even if just for a few seconds. Afterwards they are unlikely to remember the seizure and may be confused and disorientated about what has happened.

There are many causes of seizures. Any head injury or stress to the brain can cause fitting, as can brain tumours, meningitis, malaria, eclampsia in pregnancy, poisoning, lack of oxygen, raised body temperature, epilepsy, drug and alcohol use and withdrawal.

A diagnosis of epilepsy is made when someone has had at least one unprovoked seizure which cannot be attributed to any other cause.

Seizures cause rigid, out of control movements. The casualty may experience absence seizures, where they become rigid and unresponsive, full thrashing-around tonic-clonic fits, or anything in between.

Absence seizures

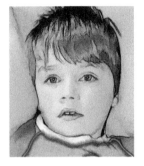

Absence seizures are relatively common in children. Initially, they may appear vague and not to be concentrating, their school performance may go down and they may appear confused as to what is happening. Further investigation by a medical specialist may show that they are having blank sessions of a few seconds repeatedly during the day. They will usually grow out of these type of seizures, but may require medication to control them.

What you might see

Sudden blank 'switch off' the child is staring into space and not responding to your voice. Sometimes the eyes roll or flicker and they can make lip smacking noises with their mouth.

What you should do

- Calmly sit them down and ensure that they are safe.
- Speak calmly and reassuringly to them and stay with them.
- Make an appointment with your family doctor and explain what happened to initiate further investigations.

Tonic-clonic fits and generalised seizures.

What might happen:

Tonic phase – they collapse to the ground as they lose consciousness. The body goes stiff and rigid and they may cry out as if in pain. This is due to an involuntary action as the muscles force air out of the lungs, the casualty is not in pain and is usually unaware of the noise they are making. They can begin to appear blue around their mouth and finger tips.

Clonic phase – they rigidly jerk around as the muscles alternately relax and tighten. They may make a snoring noise as the tongue flops to the back of the airway. They may be incontinent and could bite their tongue.

Post-Ictal phase – (a medical word meaning after a seizure). Once the jerking stops, they may be confused, sleepy, agitated or unresponsive (If you are worried about their airway put them into the recovery position). They may not know who they or you are and it could take a few minutes for it all to piece back together.

Help for a generalised seizure

- Make sure they are safe. Ease them to the ground if they are on a chair.

- Protect their head without restraining them.

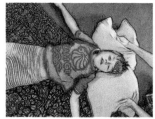

- Make a note of the time the seizure started and of the different phases – be as detailed as you can as this is extremely useful to the medical team when investigating causes and instigating treatment. Specific information as to whether one side of the body is more affected than the other can give the clinician help with their diagnosis.

- Loosen any tight clothes.

- Remove any objects they could hurt themselves against.

- Ask bystanders to move away and protect the casualty's dignity.

- Once the seizure has stopped, check the airway and breathing and place in the recovery position if unresponsive.

- Stay with the casualty and talk to them reassuringly throughout the seizure.

Phone for an ambulance:

- if it is their first seizure

- if the seizure lasts for more 5 minutes

- if they have another seizure straight after

- if they are injured

- if they are known to have seizures and this one is different.
- if you are worried at all.
- if unresponsive for more than 5 minutes after the seizure.

- Never put your fingers or anything in their mouth to try and prevent them biting their tongue – as this will cause serious injury.
- Do not try and move them unless they are in immediate danger.
- Do not restrain their movements while they are fitting.
- Do not give them anything at all to eat and drink until fully recovered.
- Never try to bring them round.

Febrile convulsions

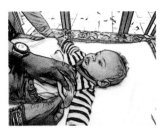

Febrile convulsions occur in young children when there is a rapid increase in their body temperature, which causes them to fit. It is fairly remarkably common, occurring in around 1 in 50 children under five years.

Bringing a child's core temperature down to prevent a seizure

Take the child's temperature. If it is higher than normal, you can help them to reduce their temperature by:

- taking off excess clothes.
- gently sponging your child under the arms and on their forehead, providing it does not cause them any distress and does not over-cool them.
- giving them plenty to drink.
- giving them paediatric paracetamol or paediatric ibuprofen to bring their temperature down and help them feel better.

Do not give your child a bath if they have a raised temperature as if they were to fit in the bath this could be dangerous for them.

If your child starts fitting:

- Move things away from them to avoid injury. Protect their head, but do not pick them up or restrain them.

- Time how long the fit lasts and observe any events during the seizure.

- Do not put anything in their mouth. They may bite their lips or tongue, but there is nothing you can do during the fit.

- Cool them down during the fit if it is possible to do so.

The fit can last from seconds to minutes, and they may go blue and stop breathing for less than a minute during this fitting period.

Once the seizure stops, they are likely to be confused and drowsy. They may be unresponsive for a while and need to be put into the recovery position. If they start fitting, move things clear to keep them safe and protect their head. Time the seizure.

Emergency services should always be called if it is someone's first fit or if you are concerned about them in any way.

If a child is known to have seizures and you and the parent are confident managing them, the paramedics may not always be necessary. However, the emergency services should be called if the convulsion lasts for more than 5 minutes, or they remain unresponsive 5 minutes after the seizure.

Unfortunately, once they have had one fit, they are likely to have more, so always keep their temperature down during illness. Fortunately, febrile convulsions do not appear to cause any long-term damage and your child will grow out of them, usually by the time they are 5 or 6 years old.

Epilepsy

A diagnosis of epilepsy is made if someone has one or more seizure without anyknown cause. The management of an epileptic fit is exactly the same as managin any other fit.

The person experiencing the fit may have an aura (a sound, taste, smell, sensation) in advance of the fit that they recognise as a sign that they are about to have a seizure and this can give them sufficient warning to get themselves onto the floor and alert someone. Usually their seizures will follow a similar pattern.

The casualty will usually be on anti-convulsant medication which can have very unpleasant side effects for them. Teachers and child carers should be aware that this medication can be quite difficult for some people to tolerate and can give children severe stomach cramps and diarrhoea as well as other unpleasant side effects.

Extremes of body temperature

Normal body temperature is between 36.5°C and 37.5°C.

Babies and the elderly find it harder to control their body temperatures and both are particularly susceptible to heat exhaustion or hypothermia. It is important that those looking after them ensure that they are wrapped up warm enough in the cold and remain well hydrated in the heat.

Heat exhaustion

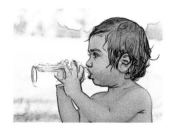

Heat exhaustion is typically caused when someone has been out on a hot day, doing some form of exercise and they have not drunk enough fluids. It is caused by a loss of salt and water through excessive sweating without rehydration.

Signs and symptoms

- Hot to touch
- Flushed or pale
- Nauseous
- Stomach cramps
- Shivery and a bit confused
- Sweaty

Treatment

- Remove excess clothing and move them to a cool place.

- Sit them down, or possibly lay them down with their legs slightly raised.

- Encourage them to rehydrate. A sports drink is a good option, or a rehydration solution such as Dioralyte - they should take regular small sips.

- Ice lollies are also helpful to cool and rehydrate them.

- Paracetamol can help.

- If symptoms get worse, get medical help.

Heat Stroke

Heat stroke is a very serious condition when the body's temperature control mechanism fails and their temperature keeps rising to dangerously high levels - beyond 40°C. The signs and symptoms are:

- High temperature

- Flushed, dry, hot skin (no sweating)

- Severe, throbbing headache

- Dizziness and sickness

- Confusion and restlessness

Treatment

- Cool the casualty down swiftly.

- Wrap them in a cold, wet sheet until their temperature falls below 38°C. This can then be replaced with a dry sheet.

- Be prepared to treat a febrile convulsion should they start fitting.

- Phone the emergency services.

Hypothermia and frostbite

Hypothermia is defined as the point at which the core body temperature falls below 35°C.

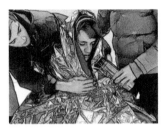

Small children and babies are particularly at risk as their temperature control area in the brain is not always fully developed. If they are out in cold conditions with insufficient warm clothing, they can quickly develop mild hypothermia.

- Elderly people also often suffer from hypothermia.

- Cold water and wet clothing brings the temperature down very fast.

- People with high levels of alcohol and drugs in their system find it harder to maintain their body temperature.

The signs and symptoms

- Pale and quiet and cold to touch.

- Shivery and then stiff with cold.

- As hypothermia develops further, they become confused, disorientated and then may lose consciousness. Severe hypothermia kills.

Treatment

- Remove cold, wet clothing and put on warm, dry clothing. Cover their head as well.

- Wrap up warm in coats and blankets, and increase the room temperature if possible.

- If unable to get indoors, wrap in a foil blanket and use a survival bag and shelter.

- Give warm drinks.

- Always seek medical advice - if their condition deteriorates phone the emergency services.

- If they lose consciousness and are breathing put them in the recovery position.

- If they stop breathing, do CPR.

- NOTE: if they are very cold, keep them still as the extreme cold can affect their heart and any swift movement can cause a cardiac arrest.

- Do not use hot water bottles or put the person in a bath to warm them, as this can warm them too quickly and cause burns.

For people who have been playing sport and are injured, it is particularly important that they are kept warm. They should sit on something to insulate themselves from the ground and it may be sensible to wrap them in a reflective blanket to retain their body heat and prevent them getting cold.

Frostbite

- Frostbite happens when an extremity (such as a finger, toe or ear) gets so cold that ice crystals form in the cells and destroy them.

- The casualty may develop pins and needles, tingling and then numbness in the affected area.

- The skin becomes hard and changes first to white, then to blue and finally turns black as the cells die.

- As the area is warmed, it can become hot, red and very painful.

Treatment

- Carefully remove jewellery if possible. It may need to be cut off.

- DO NOT rub the injury as this will make things worse. To stop the freezing getting worse, cup the affected area in your hands. Do not start to warm them if there is a danger of the area re-freezing. Move them indoors and start to warm them slowly by placing the affected area in warm water. Refer for medical help as soon as possible.

Chilblains happen because of dry cold. The cells do not freeze but the extremities become itchy, bluish-red in colour and become swollen. If it is not treated the casualty may develop blisters. Treatment is the same as for frostbite.

Medical conditions

Sepsis

Sepsis, which was previously known as septicaemia or blood poisoning, is a potentially life-threatening condition. It occurs when chemicals released into the bloodstream to fight an infection trigger inflammatory responses throughout the body.

Sepsis most commonly results from chest infections, urinary tract infections, peritonitis, or infected wounds, cuts or bites. Always regularly check wound sites following injuries or surgical procedures. If the wound becomes hot, itchy, swollen or red, you should seek medical advice promptly as this can be an early sign of infection. Prompt and potent antibiotics should be given to treat the infection and prevent it spreading.

Sepsis can be caused by a huge variety of different bacteria. However, most cases are due to common bacteria such as Streptococcus, E-coli, MRSA or C difficile. The word sepsis is derived from the Greek word sipsi (make rotten). Often, survivors of sepsis need amputations due to the flesh literally going rotten. Sepsis can lead to a severe drop in blood pressure and septic shock.

Although sepsis is extremely difficult to spot, there are usually clear signs that someone is becoming seriously unwell.

Signs and symptoms of sepsis

Sepsis is a serious condition that can look like flu, gastroenteritis or a chest infection.

Early sepsis can be difficult to recognise and often takes a while to diagnose, during which the casualty deteriorates rapidly. The sooner treatment is started, the better the outcome for the patient.

The Sepsis Trust highlights 6 key signs and symptoms to look out for.

Seek medical help urgently if your child develops any of the following:

- Slurred speech
- Extreme shivering or muscle pain
- Passing no urine (in a day)
- Severe breathlessness
- Feeling like they might die
- Skin mottled or discoloured

http://sepsistrust.org/

Any child who:

1. Feels abnormally cold to touch
2. Looks mottled, bluish or has very pale skin
3. Has a rash that does not fade when you press it
4. Is breathing very fast
5. Has a "fit" or convulsion
6. Is very lethargic or difficult to wake up

Might be critically ill

One or more of these? See a doctor urgently:

Call 999 and say you are worried about sepsis.

Sepsis can be hard to recognise at first as early symptoms are similar to flu and other common illnesses. Symptoms are also similar to meningitis.

Any child under 5 who:

1. Is not feeding
2. Is vomiting repeatedly
3. Hasn't had a wee or wet nappy for 12 hours

Might have sepsis

One or more of these? Get urgent medical advice and say you are worried about sepsis.

Common signs and symptoms of meningitis and sepsis.

Symptoms can appear in any order. Some may not appear at all.

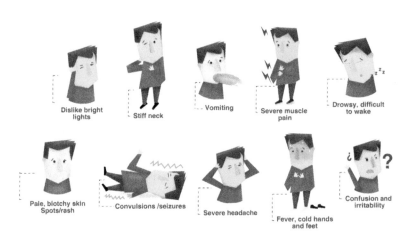

Common signs and symptoms of meningitis and sepsis in babies

Symptoms can appear in any order. Some may not appear at all.

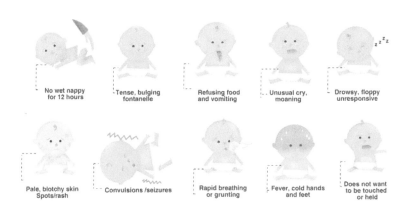

For a free copy of this poster, please email emma@firstaidforlife.org.uk

When to get urgent medical help

- If someone is getting worse and you are worried.

- If they are seriously unwell and have some of the above symptoms.

- If you are sent home from the hospital or GP surgery and the casualty is getting worse, go back. Trust your instincts and tell them why you are worried.

Meningitis

Meningitis is swelling of the meninges, the protective membranes of the brain and spinal cord. The inflammation usually results from an infection. There are various vaccination programmes to reduce the incidence of meningitis; however, even if someone has been vaccinated, they can still contract meningitis from another bacteria or virus. **Babies, toddlers and adolescents are particularly at risk.** Viral meningitis can be very unpleasant, but is rarely life threatening and most people make a full recovery. Bacterial meningitis is more serious and can be caused by a range of different bacteria. **Meningitis and septicaemia (sepsis) can be hard to recognise at first as early symptoms are similar to flu and other common illnesses. Key signs of meningitis to look out for in babies and children:**

- Pale, mottled skin.

- Cold hands and feet.

- Fever - particularly with cold hands and feet, vomiting, headache and feeling generally unwell. These early symptoms are extremely difficult to recognise as they are similar to many other milder illnesses.

- They may have a headache and in small babies the soft spot of their head (fontanelle) could be raised.

- Vomiting and diarrhoea.

- Difficulty breathing.

- Floppy, lifeless and drowsy.

- A rash which does not disappear when pressure is applied to it (the tumbler test). Never wait for the rash, as it may not appear at all.

Meningitis symptoms specific to toddlers and babies

- Refusing to eat/feed.
- Irritable, not wanting to be held/touched.
- A stiff body, with jerky movements, or floppy, unable to stand up.
- A tense or bulging soft spot on the head (fontanelle).
- A high pitched or moaning cry.

Meningitis rash and the tumbler test

With most rashes, when pressure is applied to the skin, the rash disappears. With meningitis, the rash is different and does not disappear with pressure and so can be seen when a clear glass tumbler is pressed over the skin (the tumbler test).

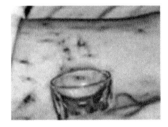

It can be harder to see a rash on dark skin, check the soles of the feet, palms of hands, roof of mouth and inside eyelids.

DO NOT WAIT FOR A RASH.

Meningitis can kill in 4 hours, so you need to take swift action.

When to call an ambulance

- IIf the baby or child is getting worse and you are seriously concerned.
- If you see a rash begin to appear and you are still able to see it if you apply pressure with the side of a glass.
- If they are seriously unwell and have some of the above symptoms.

If you are sent home from the hospital or GP surgery and the child gets worse, go back. Trust your instincts and tell them you are worried.

Diabetes

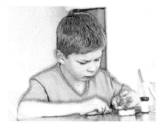

Diabetes is a condition where someone is unable to adequately regulate their blood glucose levels. The body produces the hormone insulin which helps the body to burn off the sugars that are eaten. If the body has problems with their insulin production, they will develop diabetes.

There are two types of diabetes:

Type 1 diabetes usually develops early in life and is the most common type of diabetes in children. It occurs when the body is unable to produce any insulin. Type 1 diabetes is treated with insulin injections, or by using an insulin pump.

Type 2 diabetes is the most widespread form of the condition. It tends to develop later in life, and is often linked to obesity. Type 2 diabetes develops when the body is unable to make enough insulin, or when the insulin that is produced does not work properly (known as insulin resistance). Type 2 Diabetes is controlled by diet, exercise, or oral medication - or a combination of all 3.

The first aid treatment for diabetes is more likely for low blood sugar levels than for high levels - as blood sugar can drop very quickly if the person has missed a meal or done additional exercise they hadn't anticipated.

	High blood sugar	Low blood sugar
Onset	Usually slower	Can be very quick
Levels of response	Deteriorates slowly	Can deteriorate rapidly
Skin	Dry and warm	Pale, cold and sweaty
Breathing	Deep sighing breaths	Shallow and rapid
Pulse	Rapid	Rapid
Other symptoms	Needing to wee a lot Very thirsty Hunger Pear drop smell on breath	May appear drunk

High blood sugar levels usually build over a few days or weeks, whereas lowlevels can come on very fast.

You are much more likely to be giving first aid to a diabetic patient with low blood sugar (hypo).

However, if you are looking after someone who develops weight loss, excessive urination, thirst and tiredness, these are symptoms of hyperglycaemia and they should get urgent medical attention. If they get worse and begin to get drowsy and start to lose consciousness, phone for an ambulance.

Low blood sugar/hypoglycaemia

Blood glucose levels can drop very fast if someone who is diabetic has skipped a meal, taken a lot of exercise, if they are ill, or have given themselves too much insulin. If this is not treated quickly they can rapidly start to lose consciousness and fall into a diabetic coma. This can be fatal.

Signs and symptoms of hypoglycaemia

- Behaving unusually
- May be aggressive
- Could appear slightly confused or drunk
- Turning pale, cold, shaky and sweaty
- Shallow, rapid breathing and a fast, strong pulse
- Seizures

Low blood sugar - give a sugary drink and if they feel better, follow it up with a jam sandwich or some other carbohydrate to sustain the blood sugar levels.

Treatment

- Sit them down and give them a sugary drink, or glucose sweets (not a diet drink).

- If they begin to feel better, give more drinks and some food, particularly biscuits or bread to sustain their blood sugar - a jam sandwich is great.

- If they don't feel better within 10 minutes, or they begin to get worse - phone the emergency services.

- If they lose consciousness but are breathing, put into the recovery position and phone the emergency services.

- If they stop breathing, prepare to give CPR.

Do not attempt to give an unconscious casualty anything to eat or drink. **Never** *give them insulin as this will further lower their blood sugar and could kill them.*

Even if someone appears to have recovered, ensure they receive urgent medical advice. This is particularly important at night, as insulin will still be active in the blood stream while they are asleep and the blood sugar levels will therefore drop again and they could drift from sleeping to unconsciousness.

Part 4

Useful information

What to put in your first aid kit

First aid kits need to be easily accessible in case an emergency arises. The kit should be well organised, ideally in a bag with compartments to allow you to quickly grab what you need. It is most important that the kit's contents are good quality – often cheap kit contents will not be of adequate quality.

Your kit should contain a first aid book or instructions, and contents to treat the following: major and minor bleeding, burns, breaks and sprains.

The kit should not contain medication. First aid kits for a car should be in soft padded cases or secured within the car.

The essential contents

- Tough cut scissors – strong enough to cut through clothes.

- A face shield to protect yourself when doing mouth to mouth resuscitation.

- Gloves – non sterile to protect you and sterile for treating someone with deep wounds or burns.

- Sterile medical wipes to clean a wound.

- Wound dressings of various sizes.

- Micropore tape to secure dressings and tape fingers and toes. It's also useful for labelling things.

- Calico triangular bandages are some of the most useful things in your kit, so ideally have two or more of these. Make sure they are calico, and not a cheap version made of paper.

- Sterile, non-fluffy material to stop bleeding, which can be used for slings and support bandages, are also far easier than a dressing to secure on head, knee and elbow wounds.

- Eye dressings – can also be used as small dressings for babies and toddlers.

- Sterile saline vial – for irrigating a wound, or washing grit from an eye.

- Crepe bandage – for supporting a sprain or strain.

- Plasters – for short term covering of a minor wound, (do not use for more than an hour or so as they cause wounds to become soggy).

Additional useful contents

- Burn gel or a burns dressing – to apply to a burn after cooling.

- Instant ice pack – at home you can use a bag of frozen peas. Ensure it is wrapped in a cloth before applying to skin as it can cause ice burns.

- A foil blanket to keep the casualty warm is crucially important to prevent them going into shock. They should ideally be insulated from the ground and have this wrapped round them to retain their body heat.

- Steri-strips are great to help close gaping wounds. Always get major or deep wounds swiftly seen by a medical professional.

- Sterile tweezers – for removing small splinters that can easily be grasped and pulled out in the same direction they went in (nothing else should ever be removed from a deep wound unless by a medical professional).

- AEDs – Automated External Defibrillators – available as fully or semi-automated.

- Keyring face shields – to protect yourself when resuscitating someone.

- For more detailed information as to what to put in your first aid kit please visit http://firstaidforlife.org.uk/what-put-in-first-aid-kit

Giving children medication

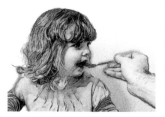

The child's parent or legal guardian should provide clear instructions about dosage and timing as well as signed and dated consent.

Medication should only be given from the original packaging and according to the doctor's original prescribing instructions.

Medication should be kept in a locked cabinet out of sight of children.

If administering to someone else's child then detailed information must be kept as to what medication was given, what dose and the exact time.

Explain to the child why they need the medicine. Tell them if it does not taste nice and have something pleasant to take the taste away.

Tip: For giving medicine in a syringe, try to keep the child as calm as possible. Hold them on your lap; it can be helpful to tuck one of their arms under yours.

Angle the syringe into the side of their cheek. Give small amounts at a time and ensure they have swallowed it all before giving any more. Do not squirt the syringe down their throat as it will frighten them and they could choke.

Tip: Giving eye drops can be very difficult. If the child keeps their eyes closed and you squeeze the drops into the outside of the eye (the other side from the tear duct), position them to allow the drops to flow across the inside of the eye and encourage them to blink a few times. This can be a lot easier than trying to get drops in with their eyes open.

How to treat an injured or unwell child

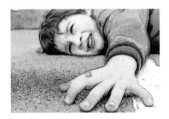

Keep calm and reassure them from their level. Examine them from the feet up, and explain all the while what you are doing.

Useful questions

- What happened?
- Where does it hurt most?
- Can you take a deep breath? This can be a distraction, but can also swiftly alert you if there is something seriously wrong.

Make the area completely safe to ensure there are no further injuries. Clean up vomit, blood or other body fluids using disposable gloves and cloths with antibacterial cleaning agents.

Have a designated bowl for vomit and ensure it is hygienically cleaned after each use and not used for anything else.

Conclusion

Thank you for taking the time to read my book.

Hopefully, you now feel confident recognising and helping with life-threatening medical emergencies as well as minor injuries. You have now equipped yourself with vital knowledge to help ensure you are never in that awful situation with someone suffering in front of you and not having a clue how to help.

This book is ideal for keeping in your loo or by your bed, so you can revisit it regularly to keep your knowledge fresh.

There will undoubtedly be updates to the information in this book and I will produce updated editions to include these. I recommend visiting our website www.firstaidforlife.org.uk which is packed full of all the latest first aid tips and advice. If you can, I would also strongly urge you to do one of our practical or online courses to consolidate these skills further and ensure your knowledge remains current.

PART 5

RESOURCES

There are many resources available for parents, child carers, and those working with children and schools.

The following are just a few that I think are particularly useful:

Potential hazards for children around the home

Kitchen	
Cooker	Don't allow saucepan handles to overhang. Oven doors may get hot. Have fire blankets and a fire extinguisher to hand.
Alcohol/medicine	Put in secure cupboards out of sight and reach
Cleaning products	Ensure the cupboard is child proof and out of reach.
Electrical appliances	Tuck away cords and don't allow them to overhang work tops.
Fridge/freezers	Large uprights might appeal as a hiding place or somewhere to explore.
Dishwasher	Never leave the tablets or powder accessible in the door of the machine.

Utility rooms	
Washing machines and tumble driers	Secure doors.
Cleaning products or chemicals	Put in locked cupboards out of sight and reach.
Buckets	Potentially a drowning risk, always empty liquids

Ironing boards & irons	Tuck away cords and don't allow them to overhang when in use – store safely when not in use or cooling.
Tools and tool boxes	Keep secure – don't leave tools out.
Carbon monoxide	Fit carbon monoxide alarms wherever there is a flame-burning appliance or open fire.

Bathroom	
Medicine/bleaches	Put in locked cupboards out of reach of hands.
Baths & showers	Use bath mats to prevent slips and falls.
Loos and toilet brushes	Secure lids down, keep brushes out of reach.
Bath time	Never leave a baby or young one unattended, ever! Run cold water first and add hot to get the right temperature. Always check the temperature yourself before putting your child in the bath. Bath thermometers can be helpful.
Hot water	Check your water temperature settings. Get thermostatic bath taps if possible, they can be helpful to prevent temperature surges.

Living areas	
Smoke alarms	Fit a smoke alarm on every level of your home and test them weekly.
Blind cords or curtain pulls	These pose a risk of strangulation. Keep out of reach and use blind clips or cordless blinds.

Furniture	May become something children climb on or up. Check for potential tipping over and secure. Don't place under windows of any height
Windows	Install window restrictors to prevent unrestricted opening
TV and appliances	Check they are secure so that they cannot fall on a child. Tuck away cables
Fires, heaters and radiators	Open fires must always be attended and a fire guard in place. Check thermostats on radiators so that they can't burn a child. Turn off heated towel rails. Use radiator covers.
Stairs	Secure carpets. Install stair gates if necessary and remove them when they begin to pose a hazard.
Highchairs	Follow the safe use instructions, always strap your child in.

Bedroom

Blind or curtain cords	These pose a risk of strangulation. Keep out of reach.
Furniture	Check safety standards. Secure in place to prevent falling on a child – for example a cupboard or drawers.
Hair straighteners and styling products	Keep well out of reach, particularly when hot or cooling

Garden & Garage

Paint and chemicals	Always store in the original containers, never decant anything. Put in locked cupboards, out of sight and reach. Dispose of anything that is not needed or if the label has become illegible.

Play equipment	Are they appropriate for their age range? Things deteriorate quickly in the open. Is it fit for use? Does it need a repair? Has it been installed safely? Empty paddling pools immediately after the activity has finished.
Pools, tubs, or spas	Fence them in or cover to prevent unsupervised access.
Plants	Remove any toxic or poisonous plants
Driveways	Ensure vision for drivers is good. Prevent child access.
Car seats	Ensure they are in the right car seat for their height, weight and age. Always strap them in safely. Activate child locks on the car.

Additional checklist for schools, nurseries, childminders and children's activity providers

The following is specific additional advice for childminders, child carers and children's activity providers.

For child-orientated businesses	
General safety	Check for trip hazards, electrical flexes or items that may fall. Check safety equipment is maintained and in date.
Doors	Are glass panels strengthened glass? Can heavy doors close on a child? Is there a secure lock on external access doors?

Hazardous items	Are plastic bags out of reach?
	Lock away chemicals or cleaning materials etc.
Water	All water activities need to be supervised.
	Check for spillage and slip hazards.
Outside	Is access secure?
Fire escape access	There needs to be adequate access/ means of escape.
	No buggies or equipment blocking access.
Ventilation and heating	Can a reasonable temperature be maintained?
	Are measures in place, such as blinds, to protect from glare and heat from sun?

Risk assessments and accident forms for schools and nurseries

Health and Safety (First Aid) regulations 1981

Employer's responsibilities

The employer has a legal obligation to ensure that there is sufficient first aid provision for the needs of the company.

- They need to consider how many and what type of first aiders are needed for their company.

- Establish what training is required to ensure they have sufficient provision and that their team of first aiders receive regular refreshers and renewals in order that they remain confident and competent in their skills.

- They need to check how many first aid kits are needed and if there is any additional equipment required.

- Ensure that staff know how and where to get first aid treatment.

Employers need to carry out a first aid needs assessment considering the following elements:

- Nature of the work and any specific workplace hazards and risks – such as chemicals, working at height, etc.
- Number of staff on site and visitors
- Organisational history concerning accidents
- Annual leave, sickness and other cover for first aid provision
- Distribution of the workforce and working patterns and shift work
- Remoteness from emergency services

Accident forms

A minor injury can lead to a major problem and so all injuries should be recorded either on a formal accident form if a business or childminder, or in a designated book if you are a nanny.

Accident books will be inspected and may be able to show trends and patterns of injuries which can lead to improvements in health and safety.

Proper accident recording can be vital written defence should there be a legal challenge concerning the accident, injury or treatment given.

An accident book is a legal document. Things written down at the time of an accident are usually considered to be more reliable evidence than things recalled from memory. The entire report should be completed in one go in the same ballpoint or non-erasable pen.

An accident record should be completed as soon as possible after the incident and should contain the following information:

- Full name of the casualty
- Casualty's occupation
- Date, time and location of the incident

- What happened – in as much detail as possible

- What injuries were sustained

- Treatment given

- Medical help sought – if any

- Witnesses – names and contact details

- Layout of area – sketch if possible

- Further action required

- Parent's signature to acknowledge that they have been informed

- Name, address, occupation and signature of the person completing the report

It is good practice to state whether someone has refused medical intervention and their reasons for this. Seek medical advice if you are unsure if they are sufficiently fully conscious and alert to be able to make this decision.

Accident books can be bought from many sources and are widely available online through the HSE.

The book needs to comply with the Data Protection Act and therefore personal records need to be removed and stored securely and a member of staff designated to be responsible for the safekeeping of accident records within a lockable cabinet.

The person who has had the accident or their legal guardian is entitled to a copy of the report. This should be copied prior to filing and they should keep a record of the accident report number.

The forms should be kept for a minimum of 3 years and for a child until 3 years after their 18th birthday to give them time to take legal action as an adult should they need to do so.

Reporting of Injuries, Diseases and Dangerous Occurrences Regulations 1995

It is the responsibility of the employer or person in charge of the premises to report the following occurrences directly to the Health and Safety Executive:

The following should be reported immediately:

- Death
- Major injuries
- Dangerous occurrences
- If someone has an incident that results in them being off work (or unable to perform full duties) for more than 3 days – this needs to be reported within 10 days
- Notifiable diseases – should be reported as soon as possible

Primary or nursery school risk assessment

Risk assessment title	
Date of risk assessment	
Risk assessment completed by	EYFS Team Leader + EYFS Team
Initial review date for assessment: (6 weeks after completion date)	
Assessment review date: (annually or sooner if required)	

- A **hazard** is anything that may cause harm, such as chemicals, electricity, working from ladders, an open drawer etc.
- The **risk** is the chance, high or low, that somebody could be harmed by these and other hazards, together with an indication of how serious the harm could be.

Extract from the statutory framework for the early years' foundation stage

It is essential that children are provided with safe and secure environments in which to interact and explore rich and diverse learning and development opportunities. Providers need to ensure that, as well as conducting formal risk assessment, they constantly reappraise both the environments and activities to which children are being exposed and make necessary adjustments to secure their safety at all times.

Outdoor and indoor spaces, furniture, equipment and toys, must be safe and suitable for their purpose.

Specific legal requirements - Risk assessment

Schools will not be required to have separate policies for the EYFS provided that the requirements are met through their policies which cover children of a statutory age.

Outings - Children must be kept safe whilst on outings.

- For each specific outing, providers must carry out a full risk assessment, which includes an assessment of required adult: child ratios.

- This assessment must take account of the nature of the outing, and consider whether it is appropriate to exceed the normal ratio requirements (as set out in this document), in accordance with providers' procedures for supervision of children on outings.

Statutory guidance to which providers should have regard

- Providers should obtain written parental permission for children to take part in outings.

- Providers should take essential records and equipment on outings, for example, contact telephone numbers for the parents of children on the outing, first aid kit, and a mobile phone.

- Records should be kept about vehicles in which children are transported, including insurance details and a list of named drivers.

- Drivers using their own transport should have adequate insurance cover.

Medicines

- Providers must implement an effective policy on administering medicines.

- The policy must include effective management systems to support individual children with medical needs.

- Providers must keep written records of all prescribed medicines administered to children, and inform parents.

- Providers must obtain prior written permission for each and every medicine from parents before any medication is given.

Specific legal requirements - Risk assessment

- The provider must conduct a risk assessment and review it regularly – at least once a year or more frequently where the need arises.

- The risk assessment must identify aspects of the environment that need to be checked on a regular basis: providers must maintain a record of these particular aspects and when and by whom they have been checked.

- Providers must determine the regularity of these checks according to their assessment of the significance of individual risks.

- The provider must take all reasonable steps to ensure that hazards to children – both indoors and outdoors – are kept to a minimum.

Statutory guidance to which providers should have regard

- The risk assessment should cover anything with which a child may come into contact.

- The premises and equipment should be clean, and providers should be aware of the requirements of health and safety legislation (including hygiene requirements).

- This should include informing and keeping adults up-to-date.

- A health and safety policy should be in place which includes procedures for identifying, reporting and dealing with accidents, hazards and faulty equipment.

References:

Accident statistics:

https://publichealthmatters.blog.gov.uk/2017/02/28/preventing-accidentsin-children-under-five/

http://www.hassandlass.org.uk/

http://www.makingthelink.net/accidents-and-child-development

https://www.gov.uk/government/news/new-reports-aim-to-help-reduceaccidents-to-children-and-young-people-in-the-home-and-on-the-roads

https://www.gov.uk/government/publications/reducing-unintentional-injuries-among-children-and-young-people

http://www.chimat.org.uk/

http://www.rospa.com/media-centre/press-office/press-releases/detail/?id=1497

http://www.drfoster.com/

Safety resources:

https://www.gov.uk/child-car-seats-the-rules

https://www.gov.uk/government/news/new-guidance-aims-to-help-prevent-unexpected-child-deaths-in-london http://www.rospa.com/home-safety/advice/product/toy-safety/

https://www.gov.uk/law-on-leaving-your-child-home-alone

http://www.riddor.gov.uk

Health and Safety Executive latest guidance on first aid training:

http://www.hse.gov.uk/firstaid/first-aid-training.htm

http://www.hse.gov.uk/pubns/priced/l74.pdf

http://www.hse.gov.uk/firstaid/legislation.htm#duties

Brake Road Safety Charity -

http://www.brake.org.uk/

Children's' Activities Association

http://www.childrensactivitiesassociation.org/

AED Signage -

https://www.resus.org.uk/pages/AEDsign.htm

School and nursery resources:

http://www.hse.gov.uk/firstaid/faqs.htm#first-aid-in-schools

https://www.gov.uk/government/publications/
supporting-pupils-at-school-with-medical-conditions--3

https://www.gov.uk/health-safety-school-children

Resources for medical conditions:

The Resuscitation Council guidelines - https://www.resus.org.uk/

ERC guidelines - https://www.erc.edu/

St John and the Red Cross 10th Edition

Sudden Infant Death Syndrome - www.lullabytrust.org.uk

Sudden cardiac death - http://www.c-r-y.org.uk/sudden-cardiac-death/

British Heart Foundation

http://www.asthma.org.uk/

Anaphylaxis Trust

http://www.youtube.com/watch?v=CjgbwmQy2r8 - how to use a Jext

http://www.youtube.com/watch?v=pgvnt8YA7r8 - how to use an Epipen

Poisons database

http://www.npis.org/toxbase.html

Head injuries in sport - http://www.englandrugby.com/my-rugby/players/
player-health/concussion-headcase/

Headway brain injury https://www.headway.org.uk/

Epilepsy

http://www.epilepsy.org.uk/info/seizures/febrile-convulsions

Great Ormond Street Hospital advice on febrile convulsions:

http://www.gosh.nhs.uk/parents-and-visitors/
general-health-advice/a-z-child-health/febrile-convulsions/

http://www.mayoclinic.org/diseases-conditions/sepsis/home/ovc-20169784

Sepsis Trust - http://sepsistrust.org/info-for-the-public/

Meningitis Research Foundation -

http://www.diabetes.org.uk/

A specific website designed for children with diabetes - http://www.diabetes.org.
uk/Guide-to-diabetes/My-life/

child accident
prevention trust

One Step A

I might FALL...

0-3 months
...when you carry me.
Clear toys away so
you don't trip.

0-9 months
...if I roll off the
Change my n
on the floor.

I might SUFFOCATE or get STRANGLED...

0-12 months
...in duvets and pillows.
Don't use them on my bed.

I might get POISONED...

7-24 months (and over)
...if I put medicines in my mouth.
Put them out of my reach.

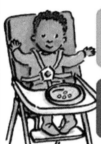

I might DROWN...

0-24 mo
...in only 5 d
Don't lea

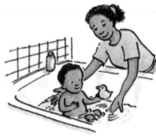

I might CHOKE...

0-8 mo
...if you p
Hold m

I might get BURNT...

0-18 months
...on hot drinks.
Put me down before
you pick up yours.

0-24 months (an
...if you put hot water
the bath first.
Always put the col

This chart shows
you when you
need to begin to
think about risks
for children
0-24 months.

We might have a FIRE...

Check our smoke alarms are work

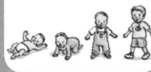

Birth ⟶ 3 months
• I can lift my head.
• I can wriggle and kick.

5 months ⟶ 8
• I can roll over, reach for
put things in my mouth.
• I can crawl, open and sh
sit up on my own.

© Child Accident Prevention Trust 2009 CH002

Remembe

d : keeping your child safe at home (0-24 months)

6-24 months (and over)
...from my highchair or pram. Use a five point harness.
...if I climb the stairs. Use safety gates.
...out of the window. Move things I might climb on away.
...out of my cot if I climb on my cot toys. Take big toys out.

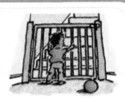

10-24 months (and over)
...on blind or curtain cords.
Tie up blind or curtain cords so there's no hanging loop.

months (and over)
nk cleaning products.
them out of reach and sight,
locked away.

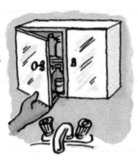

bath.

10-24 months (and over)
...in garden ponds or paddling pools.
Don't leave me alone near them.

6-24 months (and over)
...on food that's too big or an odd shape. **Please cut it up small.**
...on small objects, like coins. **Keep them out of my reach.**

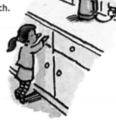

4-24 months (and over)
...if I touch your hot hair
straighteners. Keep them
and irons out of my reach.

7-24 months (and over)
...if I grab hot drinks,
pots or kettles.
Keep them out of my reach.

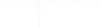

**Plan how we'll escape in a fire and
practise what we should do.**

onths → 10 months	11 months → 13 months	18 months → 24 months
can pick up small things and pull yself up to stand now.	• If you hide something from me I still know it's there.	• I like to be like you and do what you do.
can walk if I hold onto the furniture nd may be able to climb.	• I can walk all by myself.	• I can unscrew lids now.

ildren do the same things at each age

www.capt.org.uk

Poster available to order from www.capt.org.uk

I do hope this information has been useful to you.

There is no better way to learn first aid than joining one of our award-winning practical or online first aid courses.

Please visit www.firstaidforlife.org.uk and www.onlinefirstaid.com for more information and loads of free resources. You can also sign up to receive updates.

Learn pet first aid with us at www.firstaidforpets.net.

For further information or to ask me any questions, please email me:

emma@firstaidforlife.org.uk

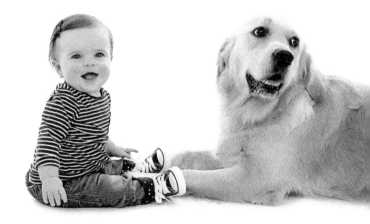

Lightning Source UK Ltd.
Milton Keynes UK
UKOW07f0351270417
300016UK00012B/69/P

9 780995 490031